Vitality Fusion

A Comparative, Interactive Survey of
Western, Chinese and Ayurvedic Medicine

SUSAN SHANE, L.AC.

"**I have been a health practitioner** *and teacher of health practitioners for over 35 years. I have taught thousands of doctors, and I came to a point where I could quickly profile which of my students would be successful, and who would not. Dr. Susan Shane is one of those students who still remains in my memory. She remains in my memory because of her intelligence, grace, compassion, and clarity......all qualities needed to succeed in the healing profession.*

I am proud to have had Dr. Shane as a student, and I am even prouder to have her as a colleague. I eagerly await her new book. Knowing Dr. Shane the way I do, I look forward to her book succeeding to further illuminate the healing landscape."

-DR. STEPHEN STITELER, LOS ANGELES, CA

"**I was trained as a Molecular Biologist** *and worked on Cancer Research for more than 13 years, so I came from a very rational world, where the brain rules everything. Fortunately, today's Medicine is not only focused on treating our physical body. So many medical studies have shown the importance of our emotional body. We have to release our negative emotions such as anger, resentment and sadness so our heart can embrace and share love.*

Acupuncture is a powerful tool, it helps us to release that negativity so we can connect to our Heart and let go of all the blockages. Being able to let go is difficult, but people like Susan are a real gift. Susan is a wonderful healer; she shares more than her knowledge of acupuncture. Her healing session goes beyond that.

Our physical body communicates to us every moment and it has beautiful lessons to teach us only if we are willing to listen. If we ignore the messages of our physical body and don't release our negative emotions then serious illness can happen. I hope that this book will help you to experience this happiness in your heart."

-NATHALIE BRUEY-SEDANO, PH.D.

"**Susan utilizes a multidimensional, intuitive approach** *to her patients' acupuncture treatment. She is very insightful and takes the time to give clear explanations of the treatment's meaning and importance. Susan facilitates her patients' healing by sharing her insights with them to deepen their understanding of the interconnections between their health and specific mind-body-spirit issues they may be dealing with."*

-PAM CERECK, SENIOR STAFF SOFTWARE ENGINEER

"**Fourteen years ago, I met Susan** and had my first acupuncture treatment. At that time in my life, I was accustomed to being bedridden with a bronchitis-like illness on a regular schedule of three times a year. We started the treatment on the day my symptoms became noticeable. During the treatment, I started to feel better and I have never had the same health issue since. From this experience, I began to trust other methods of healing that were different from what I had always known. I have returned to acupuncture treatments for a wide variety of health issues from concerns related to the female experience to emotional issues to bacterial and viral illness. Acupuncture treatments are a central part of the ongoing health maintenance schedule that I keep in order to be ready for whatever life throws at me."

-HEATHER DOTY, SAN DIEGO, CA

"**I first met Susan Shane in 1997,** fourteen years ago. I had been battling fibromyalgia, diagnosed eight years earlier, but suddenly I began experiencing constant pain in my right wrist combined with a loss of dexterity in my hand. After running a nine-month gauntlet of doctors' and chiropractors' appointments, wrist and thumb braces, and cortisone shots, I was finally referred to Susan for acupuncture treatments. After three weeks of treatments with Susan, the hand and wrist pain was gone, and I could again button my blouses, lift heavier objects, and unscrew jar lids! I have been seeing Susan once a month ever since.

I have learned so much from her, not only about the management of my fibromyalgia, but also about Eastern medicine and how one's spiritual and mental health affects one's physical well-being as well. Susan has done more than just administer treatments; she has recommended reading materials; suggested exercises; proposed homework assignments; and just generally offered valuable encouragement and advice in dealing with my problems. Susan and acupuncture have been a Godsend to me. I highly recommend both!"

-RITA MCCARTHY, TEMECULA, CA

"**My husband and I wanted more than anything to start a family,** but we were having difficulty conceiving. The fertility doctors were unable to help and said it just might not happen for me. That's when I sought help from Susan Shane. Her approach involving acupuncture, herbal supplements, and an improved relationship between my body and food and nutrition created a physical, mental and spiritual state that allowed me to conceive. I am now the mother of two beautiful children!"

-JAIME MICKEY, SAN LUIS OBISPO, CA

This book is not intended to replace the services of any type of medical healthcare provider in the diagnosis or treatment of illness or disease. Any application of the material set forth in the following pages is at the reader's discretion and sole responsibility. In addition, while links to any related material contained within the book may be updated from time to time, no representation can be made that such links will remain active.

ISBN 978-0-09853914-3-0

Front Cover Description:
The central image represents heaven, man and earth: the circle is heaven, the body outline is man and the square is earth. The Chinese characters, starting from the top and moving in a clockwise direction, are the elements fire, earth, metal, water and wood. The colored circles along the mid line of the body represent chakras, or energy centers of the body.

Acknowledgements

I thank God for the strength and guidance I received in completing this project. My beautiful family has been supportive and insightful throughout this journey, and I am truly grateful for their help, especially my husband, Michael Nicita: without his creativity, publishing and technical expertise, this book, in any of its various formats, would not have been possible. I am also thankful to my daughter Sarah Nicita, and Tom Hunter, for their illustrations and artwork, to Clearstory and Fabrizio Scippa Grafica for their design and illustration contributions, and to my son, Alexander, for his suggestions about the book's history chapter.

My mentors, Dr. Yitian Ni, Dr. Stephen Stiteler, Diane Sall and Dianna C. Gregg, have also provided encouragement and support. In the early stages of creating this book, the following people had been very instrumental in caring for and guiding me: Toby Rafelson, Bob Rafelson, Gail Randazzo, Elly and Jack Nadel, Miriam Bass, Sheila Ostrow, Fonda St. Paul, Susan Ross, Cliff Lachman, Natalie Cole, Dr. Lillian Glass, Sherry Robb and Renee Golden.

If I were to try to distill my inspiration for *Vitality Fusion* down to the influence of a single person, however, that person would be my dear friend, Liz Helton, who now watches over me as she dances with the angels in heaven.

Table of Contents

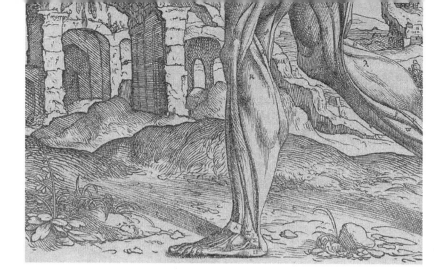

Introduction

The search for achieving optimal health can take a lifetime. For some, the search itself becomes a way of life. Regardless of where we perceive ourselves to be on this path, it is certainly true that each of us engages in this search in different ways, stumbling across answers that are as unique as we are: what works for some of us in assisting in the attainment of that elusive healthy balance may not work at all for others.

Like the people that compose them, different cultures approach this search in different ways. Three of the most popular approaches to the concept and practice of health care in the world today are those of Western, Chinese and Ayurvedic medicine. Each type of approach has attempted, over centuries, to meet the medical needs of its respective community: each, in its own unique way, has attempted to devise methods of maintaining and bettering overall health, while at the same time developing techniques to effectively restore the health of those who are ailing.

As our world has grown smaller, especially with the widespread use of the Internet, these diverse cultures have intermingled and shared their differing perspectives. And in their search for their own personal health balance, what some of their members have discovered is that while their particular culture's form of health care may work for others, it is not appropriate for them. This has prompted research across time and national boundaries, research that has surfaced the recent cross-cultural interest in health care. This is precisely the focus of this book. The survey, synthesis and "interactive" materials the book provides will hopefully empower the reader to explore new cross-cultural paths in achieving vitality and balance in their health that is as effective as it is personal.

And though there is much material in this book that recounts the rather impersonal development of medical theory and practice in three different cultures, its message remains that very personal one. In that context, please allow me to share some personal information about my own journey to this particular point in my life as a healthcare professional.

Running, playing tag or dodge ball, climbing, spinning or just dancing around, were, for me, the best fun as a young child. Movement became very important to me: my body seemed to amplify both my voice and my joy. There was probably a deeper reason why movement became so important to me as a child: when I was not playing, I was assisting the rest of my family with many household responsibilities. I had more than a usual share because my father was paralyzed from the waist down and in a wheelchair, the result of back pain and a subsequent accident.

I have no memories of him ever walking, his paralysis started when I was two. He needed help with cooking, laundry, vacuuming and outdoor gardening chores. He had had back discomfort for many years and had multiple surgeries to treat the condition. At that time, therapeutic baths at the hospital were provided as part of the recovery regimen after a surgery. After one particular therapy bath to help his legs and back heal, an orderly decided to lift him out of the water. My father asked the orderly to get more help, because my dad realized he didn't have the strength yet to lift his own legs out of the water. The orderly didn't listen, so he attempted to do it unassisted and, unfortunately, my dad slipped through the orderly's arms. This resulted in my dad crushing his back against the tile hospital floor. He never walked again.

I truly realized at a very young age how precious my body was and why I needed to take care of it properly. We are all products of our experience, and I am certain that my childhood experiences "guided" my career toward natural medicine, and a desire to teach people about the best way to ensure their own vitality and health.

As I grew older, my interest in movement also grew: I loved sports and participated in gymnastics, dance, cheer, and track and field. I felt strong, flexible and happy when exercising and performing. This passion led me to major in dance at UCLA. One week before I started college, my dad passed away.

I started my studies at UCLA, attended Santa Rosa and Napa junior colleges for summer courses, and finished my Bachelor's degree in Theater Arts from Sonoma State University, but, before graduating, took a semester off to dance professionally in Osaka, Japan. This is where I was first introduced to the

Eastern philosophy of health. The experience changed my life. I learned to add healthy foods such as sushi, sweet potatoes, miso soup and chestnuts into my diet. I tried Japanese acupressure for the first time, to deal with the rigors of dancing and to keep my body in optimal shape. The doctor who gave the acupressure treatments gave me a present on my first visit: it was a book entitled *Japanese Finger-Pressure Therapy Shiatsu* by Tokujiro Namikoshi. This was the perfect gift; just how perfect was something I didn't realize at the time – that would come later as I began to study both Swedish massage and Chinese medicine. I noticed in Osaka that elderly people were healthy and walking easily throughout the town. They knew how to take care of their bodies, and, I thought to myself, I wanted to be that vital as I aged.

Upon graduation, I decided to pursue a dance career in Los Angeles. I enjoyed training and performing in shows and a few dance videos. One of the more interesting highlights was being part of the national touring Sesame Street show (my character was both a Keystone Cop and, in a rather strange bit of foreshadowing, the Lady Doctor). We travelled by bus and during those long rides, I would read books about anatomy and kinesiology. I couldn't stop reading and learning. When I returned back to Los Angeles from the show, I realized that I was more interested in learning about health and the body than performing as a dancer. As my interests began to shift, I was unexpectedly approached at one of my favorite dance studios by some individuals in the waiting area, who asked me if I wanted to teach them to exercise. Within a week, I had a few clients and my private health and fitness training company, Shape by Shane, was born.

People enjoyed the fitness training and so did I. Teaching people how to breathe, move with proper awareness and alignment, and accomplish their personal fitness goals were all sources of great satisfaction for me. (One wonderful perk to this job was that I travelled around the country with my clients if they needed my assistance.) This turned out to be only the beginning of my healthcare journey. I continued my education by learning the

Gold's Gym body-building program, Swedish massage, Reiki energy massage and earning a masters degree in Traditional Chinese Medicine. In the process, I was fortunate enough to be interviewed by the national Financial News Network, or FNN, American Entrepreneur program as well as the magazines *New Body, Men's Guide to Fitness* and *Mature Health*.

After becoming a licensed acupuncturist, both nationally and in California, I left Los Angeles and moved to New York, for a short while, finally settling in San Diego. I opened two acupuncture offices and began to incorporate all the various health information at my disposal to help support my clients. During this time, I volunteered at Deepak Chopra's Center for Mind Body Medicine at the L'Auberge Inn in Del Mar. My job was to assist the executive secretary, Rose Murphy, with her administrative needs. It was requested that I read Deepak Chopra's *The Seven Spiritual Laws of Success* and *Perfect Health*. Just as my acupuncture interest began with a book, it was these books that first sparked my continuing interest in Ayurvedic medicine.

My career went on to include health and wellness lectures and presentations at corporations and college campuses, post graduate studies with Dr. Yitian Ni in gynecology and a seat on the Community Board of Advisors at the Scripp's Center for Integrative Medicine, a position I held for eight and a half years.

San Diego is also where I began my family. While pregnant, I was especially careful to eat and sleep well, surround myself with a positive environment, and listen very carefully to my growing bodies' needs. I would journal to focus this listening. I played lots of classical music and received acupuncture to keep me and the baby strong and healthy. Both of these things continued through the labor: my husband took care of the music and my Chinese medicine teacher and mentor, Dr. Yitian Ni, administered acupuncture and acupressure. By taking care of myself and creating a beautiful environment, my pregnancies resulted in the delivery of two healthy babies.

I kept practicing as an acupuncturist as my children grew, but downsized my practice. I couldn't stop working, completely, because I still wanted to help people to be healthy. To expand my life skills and to develop new exercise techniques to share with clients, I studied taekwondo, and am currently a second-degree black belt. For the same reasons, I wanted to learn more about tai qi, and so travelled to China, and studied at Chenjiagou, the birthplace of taiqichuan.

At some point in this personal journey, my interests fused with the need to share what I had learned in a way that might reach more people than my current practice would allow. It is my hope that this book accomplishes that purpose. It attempts to provide a survey of each of the three main approaches to restoring and maintaining optimal health, while at the same time allowing for personalization of this wisdom. This is the purpose of the exercises at the end of each chapter. Chapter Five, which treats exercise, has an especially important follow-up to the cultural survey, as it introduces an exercise program I have used for many years, one that I have named *Exaircise*. A brief summary of each of the chapters follows.

Chapter One begins with a historical perspective of the three medical disciplines. This chapter further explores the unique schools of thought that each has developed, with an emphasis on the written works that form the "textbooks" with which their physicians have traditionally been trained. This chapter also shows the differences and similarities of the three disciplines as they have evolved over the years into the types of medical practices we see today, including comparative timelines highlighting key historical events.

Chapter Two looks at the anatomical, philosophical, diagnostic and treatment principles upon which Western, Chinese and Ayurvedic medicine have been based. The viewpoints of each are defined, explained and compared. In deference to the very personal nature of each of our own journeys toward health, a medical questionnaire is provided at the end of the chapter. The reader is encouraged to begin to compile a personal health profile that will be further defined in discussions in subsequent chapters.

Chapter Three discusses the development of herbs and pharmaceuticals as they apply to the treatment and care of ailments. Given the breadth of the work available from each of the three disciplines in this area, only a relatively cursory description of similarities and differences is provided. A personal drug and herb diary is provided at the end of this chapter.

Chapter Four outlines the different approaches of the three medical disciplines to the basics of good nutrition and the need for energizing the body with the selection of the proper foods. The process of digestion and metabolism are explained as they relate to the types of foods we eat. The role protein, carbohydrates, fats, fibers, vitamins, minerals and water place are explored. This chapter explains how Chinese medicine utilizes tastes, temperatures, elements of nature, organ analysis and seasonal climate changes to determine nutrition needs. The influence of the doshas or Ayurvedic body types, nature's four seasons, food tastes and textures depicts how Ayurvedic medicine makes nutrition decisions. This chapter also includes a food plate used in the West to illustrate healthy eating choices. Again, the reader is asked to complete a food diary to record daily eating habits.

Chapter Five provides an illustrated survey of Western, Chinese and Ayurvedic body typing and ideologies. This chapter also introduces a special exercise program called Exaircise, that utilizes the highlights from each of these disciplines to strengthen the lower back. A fitness diary and measurement chart are included for charting progress for these and other exercises drawn from each discipline, and a muscular body chart is provided for quick reference.

Chapter Six introduces the concept that our mind and body have a direct link to the level of health we experience. Some of the disciplines that support the mind and body connection are rolfing, hellerwork, dominant and non-dominant handwriting and psychoneuroimmunology. A mindbody chart is included for quick reference and a journaling exercise to experience the direct communication between the mind and the body is provided.

Chapter Seven discusses the mind, body and spirit connection. Homeopathy, naturopathy, massage, aromatherapy, color and music therapy are just a few of the health modalities examined in this chapter. It also reviews how taste, touch, smell, sight and sound therapies can influence our bodies toward greater health.

Enjoy the journey of learning and living in better health through the cross-cultural exploration that this book provides. It has been designed not just as a study of three medical disciplines but as a personal, interactive guidebook filled with nutritional guidelines, simple exercises, easy-to-use diaries and quick reference charts. If it makes your own search for achieving vitality and balance in your health just a bit easier, then it would have certainly accomplished its primary goal.

Be well,
Susan Shane
SAN DIEGO, 2012

Chapter One:
History of Western, Chinese and Ayurvedic Medicines

" If you want to understand today, you have to search yesterday."
- PEARL BUCK

Any comparison of today's three major approaches to sustaining and restoring health - the Western, Chinese and Ayurvedic medical models – necessarily begins with a search for their roots in yesterday. We will explore the development of Western medicine from its earliest origins and afterwards move to Asia for similar surveys of Chinese and Ayurvedic medicine. But, before we examine their separate histories, let's briefly look at their common prehistoric roots.

In prehistoric times, we now believe that the generally accepted "health model" was that evil spirits would enter the body and cause disease. The tribal medicine man or "first physician" would need to soothe the angry spirits to restore health. For example, if a person had severe head pain, the shaman or tribal priest used a stone instrument to cut a hole through that person's skull. This technique was called trephining and is considered the first known surgery. Today, if necessary, surgery that drills a small hole through the skull can still be used to relieve swelling and pressure on the brain. Another example of prehistoric medical practices involved providing headache relief through the ingestion of parts of the herbal tree or shrub, willow bark. We understand today that willow bark contains salicin, which is related to salicylates, which, in turn, are currently used in making aspirin. These two approaches – of looking to the environment outside the body for remedies and looking within the body itself to restore proper function – are approaches that will resonate throughout the cross-cultural surveys that follow. Even the spiritual dimension of healing, adopted by prehistoric "physicians," will echo down through the centuries in the thinking and practice of future medical models.

Part I: History of Western Medicine

Around 3000 BCE, one of the greatest civilizations of all time, that of ancient Egypt, created unique solutions to the medical questions of the day. This medical progress was codified. The first physician, Imhotep, lived during this time: he was not only a doctor, but an architect and engineer as well, designing the pyramid known as the Step Pyramid of Saqqarah. Two thousand years later, his status was raised to that of a deity and he became the god of Egyptian medicine and healing.

Other physicians started to specialize in their care, choosing, for example to specialize in internal diseases, eyes or teeth. Surgeons even wrote about how to treat dislocated or fractured bones, internal abscesses, tumors, ulcers and wounds. Two important writings, the *Ebers* and the *Smith papyri*, were compiled. The *Ebers papyrus* included specific incarnations for certain illnesses, case histories, and prescriptions such as castor oil as a cathartic and tannic acid for burns. The *Smith papyrus* contained pertinent surgical information such as compression for stopping bleeding and information about eyes, the heart and other internal organ disease. This papyrus, similar to Western medicine today,

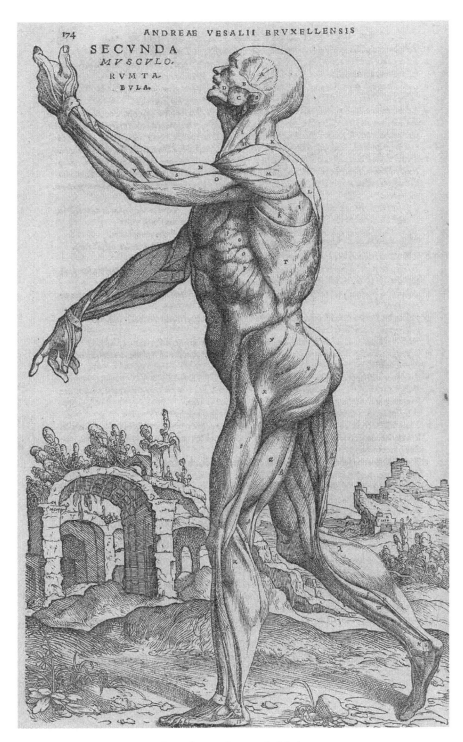

ILLUSTRATION FROM VESALIUS'S *De humani corporis fabrica*, P174, WIKIMEDIA COMMONS described what appeared upon examination to the physician, defined symptoms, identified the diagnosis, suggested therapy, and offered a prognosis.

Science and learning flourished even further under Babylon's greatest king, Hammurabi, around 2000 BCE. Medical laws defined what the physician would treat, what the physician would charge for services and what the punishment would be for the physician if there was malpractice. These regulations were inscribed on a stone pillar called the Code of Hammurabi.

Around 1200 to 600 BCE, the Hebrew civilization enforced effective techniques for preventative medicine as prescribed in the *Torah*, and in the rabbinic laws and ethics of the *Talmud*. For example, the Hebrews required isolation for people suffering with gonorrhoea, leprosy and other contagious diseases. Also, there was strong emphasis placed on public health and sanitation by prohibiting contamination of public wells and eating of contaminated foods that might carry disease.

Pythagoras, an important Greek philosopher and mathematician, is believed to have travelled the world starting around 540 BCE. He left the island of Samos, and was instructed to visit Egypt to study math, music and astronomy. Around 525 BCE, the King of Persia invaded Egypt and caused Pythagoras to relocate to Babylon. He continued his studies there and around 520 BCE left Babylon and went to India. In India, he studied the wisdom that Buddha had taught his people. Pythagoras' insights and teachings, gleaned from his many travels, influenced many cultures throughout the world, but none more than that of his native Greece, the next ascendant civilization of the ancient world. Around 400 BCE, another famous Greek, Hippocrates, showed that disease had natural causes and thus compelled many to begin to consider medicine a science and art unrelated to the practice of religion. He is believed to help write and define a code of ethics and ideals for physicians to follow while practicing medicine, called the Hippocratic Oath. The beginning of the Oath required the physician to vow to Apollo, the sun god, to Aesculapius, the god of medicine and healing, to Hygieia, the health goddess and to Panacea, the goddess of cures, that the physician would do no harm to their patient. In addition, the physician truly worked for the health of the patient and not for personal gain. The physician observed the patient using sight, taste, touch, hearing and smell to diagnose, and developed an understanding that diet, environment and personal stressors contributed to disease. The physician recommended treatment using nutrition and surgery if necessary. While this practical progress was being made, and medicine was moving into the realm of the sciences, the Greek people still worshipped Apollo and Aesculapius at temples for spiritual cures.

Aristotle, a teacher of Alexander the Great and student of Plato, emphasized the importance of the scientific method. Here, careful observation of animals and insects was recommended, and experiments incorporating dissection and studying the cause and effect of disease were suggested for greater insight and knowledge. Aristotle also described the human body as being composed of four elements manifesting as humors. These elements and humors were fire (yellow bile), earth (black bile), water (water) and air (phlegm), and they were always trying to balance each other.

The next important Western civilization that helped develop new standards in the quality of health care was the Roman Empire. The Romans had conquered Greece and Egypt by this time and incorporated their medical advancements into Rome's medical knowledge. To their own credit, the Romans made great progress improving public health. They built aqueducts that brought fresh water to Rome every day and also built excellent sewer systems.

Galen was a significant physician during this time because he performed scientific experiments on animals and developed medical theories based on these experiments. He also supported Aristotle's belief that the human body was made up of four humors. Another important physician was Celsus. He wrote encyclopedias about various diseases that included therapeutic solutions using diet, drugs and manipulation. He discussed surgery and operations for conditions such as hernias, goiter, bladder stones and cataracts. He also suggested treating fractures with splints.

Celsus' work had a profound impact on scientific thought and became popular during the latter part of the Middle Ages.

During the Middle Ages, it was the Islamic Empire that contributed to the Western world's growing corpus of medical knowledge. Rhazes, a Persian doctor, accurately described measles and smallpox. Avicenna, an Arab doctor, wrote an encyclopedia describing meningitis, tetanus and other diseases. Avicenna's information became popular in Europe for the next six hundred years. Hospitals were also established during this time and focused on studying science, teaching and provided social service.

Hospitals with medical universities also developed in Europe. The first medical school was founded in Salerno, Italy and accelerated the pace of medical learning. Christians founded charitable hospitals to aid those with leprosy. For full recovery, the religious approach held that it was also necessary to cure the soul. Scientific examination was not preferred except for Aristotle and Galen's prescriptions because they integrated science with religious practices and thought. Outbreaks of leprosy were significant but when the bubonic plague, or Black Death, traversed through Europe, it killed one-fourth of its population. After this tragedy, the development and advancement of public health became priority.

Public hospitals were built during the Renaissance era. Another important focus during this revolutionary time was on human dissection, a scientific approach that allowed for a better understanding of human anatomy. Leonardo da Vinci recorded his anatomical findings in over 750 drawings. Andrea Vesalius, a doctor and university professor, also performed many dissections.

He wrote the first human anatomy book called *On the Fabric of the Human Body* in 1543. This book replaced the information provided by Galen and Avicenna. A French physician, Ambroise Pare, became the "father of modern surgery." He developed a mild ointment for topical use on infections rather than using burning oil to disinfect, which allowed the wound to heal naturally. A Swiss doctor and "father of toxicology," Philippus Paracelsus, emphasized the importance of understanding drug chemistry since each ingredient interacts and effects the other. He believed that disease came from outside the body and that the correct chemical configuration cured the body. This was contrary to how Aristotle and Galen approached healing the body with balancing the four elements and humors.

Discovering how blood circulated throughout the body improved medical care after the Renaissance. Blood circulation via the arteries and veins and the function of the heartbeat and pulse were documented in a book, *On the Motion of the Heart*, by an English physician, William Harvey, in 1628. Harvey's work directed scientists to focus on the knowledge of the body's structure to better explain how the body worked. Another great discovery during this time, considered by many to be the beginning of modern Western medicine, was made by Dutch scientist Anton van Leeuwenhoek. He invented and further developed the microscope to study micro-organisms such as bacteria, red blood cells and protozoa.

Smallpox was a contagious and lethal disease during the 1700's: either people died or were left with disfiguring, life-long scars. But, curiously, if a person somehow managed to survive smallpox, that person did not ever have smallpox again. Following the lead of this imparted immunity, doctors injected small amounts of smallpox in healthy people, with the result that some survived, and some did not. It was English physician Edward Jenner who developed a safe injection to prevent smallpox. Influenced from his understanding of Turkish inoculations, he used material from a cowpox sore and tried injecting the matter into a boy. The boy developed cowpox which was relatively harmless, and survived. Afterwards, Jenner injected the boy with material from a smallpox sore and the boy did not get smallpox: Jenner hypothesized that the boy had developed sufficient immunity from the cowpox injection. This was the first recorded vaccination. By documenting a procedure of building up resistance to a disease in order to prevent the disease, Jenner laid the groundwork for the modern science of immunology.

Also during this time, Georg Stahl, a chemist and professor of medicine, believed that the movement in all living systems resulted from a "soul presence." This theory was called animism. In addition, Paul-Joseph Barthez, a French physician, believed that all living forms had an *élan vitale* or life force. Another school of thought was proposed by Samuel Hahnemann. He believed that "like heals like" and that giving medicine which produced the same symptoms as the disease along with smaller dosages of that particular medicine would cure without harm. This system was called homeopathy.

The previous study and deciphering of the anatomy of the body allowed for a medical science curriculum to evolve in the 1800's. Clinical practice flourished. One major reason was the discovery and use of ether as an anesthetic in the 1840's. Crawford Long, an American physician, and William Morton, an American dentist, independently discovered that ether gas could be safely used during surgeries or other medical procedures. Rudolf Vichow, a German physician and scientist, examined cells and their changes under improved microscopes. This study of cellular pathology helped to explain the cause of diseases. Louis Pasteur, a French chemist, researched how microbes such as bacteria and yeast could cause disease. He also discovered how to eliminate these germs to safely preserve food and milk. Robert Koch, a German doctor, also studied microbes. He isolated micro-organisms such as anthrax to determine which organism caused a particular disease. Another important improvement occurred when Joseph Lister, an English surgeon, demonstrated how sterilizing equipment with antiseptic such as phenol, also known as carbolic acid, made surgery safer. Infections definitively decreased. Eventually doctors wore surgical masks, gloves and gowns during medical procedures to make the operating room even more hygienic.

In 1847, doctors founded the American Medical Association to improve the national medical standards. Also during the mid-1800's, nurses organized and founded their own medical profession.

With amazing discoveries and organization, medicine advanced and continued to greatly improve. In 1895, Wilhelm Roentgen, a German physicist, discovered X-rays so that the body could be seen interiorly without surgery to the patient. In 1898, Pierre and Marie Curie, French physicists, discovered radium, and fostered its use to treat tumors. In 1928, Sir Alexander Fleming, a Scottish bacteriologist, discovered the bacteria-killing mold, penicillium. A few years later, English scientists isolated and mass produced Penicillin, a product of this mold, to create the first antibiotic. Also, during the early 1900's, Christian Eijkman of the Netherlands and Frederick Hopkins from England, showed the importance of vitamins in supporting optimal health.

During the latter part of the 1900's, engineering and technological advances greatly improved medicine. For example, open heart surgery was even more successful when a heart pacemaker was installed to regulate the heartbeat. By the 1970's, CAT scans or computerized axial tomography and PET scans or positron-emission tomography appeared. In 1980, the MRI or magnetic resonance imaging arrived. Currently, rapid progress continues in robotic surgery, stem cell research, gene therapy and the use of SPECT (Single Photon Emission Computed Tomography) cameras.

Besides looking forward toward technology for new solutions to age-old questions, Western medicine has also begun to look eastward, drawing from even more ancient traditions of medical theory and practice. Let's do the same, and begin our survey with the mythological origins of Chinese medicine.

Western Medicine Timeline

8000 BCE	*trephining - first surgical treatment*
2700 BCE	**Imhotep** - *first physician*
2500 BCE	*Egyptians organized first systematic method of treating disease*
400 BCE	**Hippocrates** *emphasized disease was natural*
100 CE	**Galen** *based medical theories on scientific experiments*
900	*first medical school started in Salerno, Italy*
1543	**Versalius** *wrote first human anatomy book*
1550	**Pare** *designated as father of modern surgery*
1628	**Harvey** *discovered blood circulation*
1676	**Leeuwenhoek** *invented the microscope*
1796	**Jenner** *developed first vaccination*
1846	**Long and Morton** *discovered first anesthetic*
1850	**Vichow** *founder of cellular pathology and* **Pasteur and Koch-** *founders of microbiology*
1865	**Lister** *developed antiseptic surgery*
1895	**Roentgen** *developed X-rays*
1898	**Curies** *discovered radium*
1900	**Eijkman and Hopkins** *discovered vitamin importance*
1928	**Flemming** *discovered penicillin*

1973	*CAT scan developed*
1980	*MRI developed*
Current	*robotics, SPECT camera, gene therapy, stem cell research*

Part II: History of Chinese Medicine

The origin of Chinese medicine is steeped in both history and mythology. According to one of the popular creation myths, heaven and earth began when the legendary Pan Gu emerged from darkness and chaos. He grew so big that his body parts became mountains, rivers, the sun and moon, all things yin and yang. Pan Gu also miraculously birthed Fu Xi around the time of 3,322 BCE. Fu Xi was an enlightened hero who taught people how to fish, how to trap animals and invented calligraphy. He wrote about and described the universe in *The Book of Changes*, or *I Ching*.

Chinese medicine, both in history and myth, evolved and changed with whatever ruling power, or dynasty, governed China. This governance began with the Three Supreme and Five Rulers Dynasty lasting approximately from 2852 -2205 BCE. Shen Nong, also known as the Red Emperor or Divine Farmer, lived during this time and invented agriculture. He taught people how to cultivate the earth to grow food, but also emphasized the tasting of herbs in order to discover their medical benefits. He wrote about his findings in the *Pen T'sao* or *The Herbal*. This was the first herbal medicinal text. Another legendary sage was Huangdi, a mystical chief of a tribe from the Yellow river. He invented chariots, boats and introduced the early forms of martial arts. He was most famous for the dialogues he had with the physician, Qi Bo. These discussions were recorded in *The Yellow Emperor's Classic of Internal Medicine*, or the *Nei Jing*, the oldest Chinese medical text, itself a compendium of treatments of various medical topics.

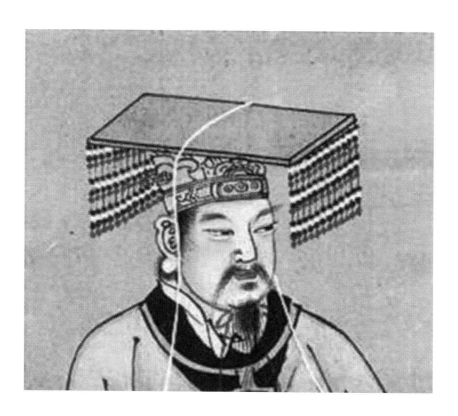

The origins of Chinese medicine continued to be shrouded in myth and legend, with this period also including the Xia Dynasty, which lasted from approximately 2100 BCE to 1600 BCE and the Shang Dynasty, which lasted from about 1600 BCE to 1046 BCE. This was a time where nature and man worked together in harmony. The primary concern was caring for the land and animals. Practicing many spiritual rituals were also a tradition. The culture was kind. Weapons as well as tools were made out of bronze, bones and stone such as jade. To keep warm, the artemesia vulgaris herb was rolled up and burned in a process that became known as moxibustion.

The next Dynasty was the Zhou Dynasty, or Golden Era, which lasted from 1045 BCE to 256 BCE. This was when Huangdi, a

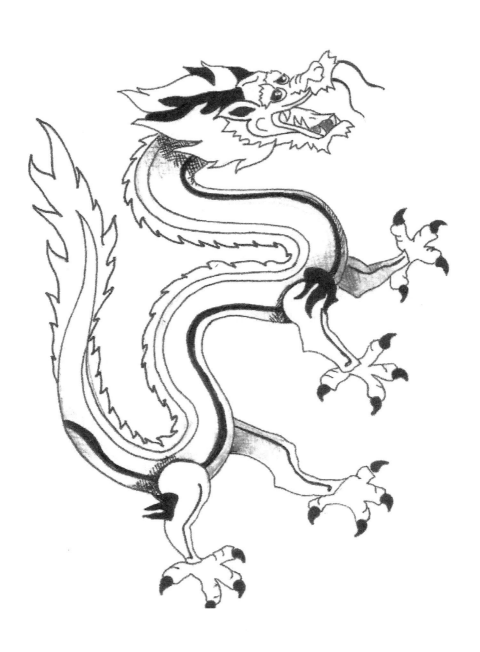

CHINESE DRAGON, ILLUSTRATED BY SARAH NICITA

famous physician, actually lived. He developed great insights into medicine, insights that eventually became part of the *Yellow Emperor's Classic of Internal Medicine*. This book contained two sections, the *Su Wen* or *Plain Questions* and the *Lingshu* or *Spiritually Changing Pivot*. Each section originally had 81 chapters. The Chinese medical information described in this valuable book included concepts that stated the creation of heaven as yang and the creation of earth as yin. Evil spirits and supernatural causes were not the only reason to be ill: natural causes such as diet, emotions and lifestyle had an impact on health and vitality. Another important text written during this era, in 651 BCE, possibly by the physician Bien Que, was *The Difficult Classic* or *Nan Jing*. This book also contained 81 chapters. Each chapter discussed one "difficult" topic of medicine. Zou Yan, a philosopher who lived from approximately 305 BCE to 240 BCE, founded a school of Naturalists and emphasized the Five Elements theory of nature.

Medicine was reaching a high level of advancement (even the government established charity hospitals) but so were literature, art, religion and government. Chuang Tzu, Lao Tzu, Confucius and Mencius, all great philosophers, lived during this time. Lao Tzu was known as the "father of Taoism," and authored the *Tao Te Ching* or *The Canon of the Tao and its Virtue*. This book described how to live harmoniously with the universe by understanding nature, taking good care of your health with moderation, and using compassion and humility when interacting with others. Buddhism highly regarded the teachings in this book. Chuang Tzu was a Taoist who emphasized living as one with nature. Confucius emphasized ethical social relations with just and sincere conduct towards others and, in particular, within government. He valued the harmony and humanity of the Xia and Shang dynasties. Mencius was a supporter of Confucianism and believed that human nature was good. Taoism and Confucianism were valued but so was Legalism: here, strict and impersonal laws were enforced by the military and wealthy authorities. Art continued with bronze work but also expanded into iron, silk and lacquer creations.

The Qin dynasty lasted from 221 BCE to 206 BCE and the Han dynasty lasted from 206 BCE to 220 CE. The Han dynasty, or Renaissance age, reflected the influence of the previously mentioned great philosophers. In particular, Confucianism dominated the practice of medicine. A Confucian doctor was trained in the classics with a strong literary emphasis. This profession was considered the greatest honor, done for personal charity and not for financial gain, though the reality was that these doctors primarily helped the wealthy. The common people were treated by folk doctors who were trained by family members or religious teachers. Two famous physicians who practiced during this time were Zhang Zhongjing and Hua To. Zhang Zhongjing wrote the *Shang Han Lun* or *Treatise on Being Affected by the Cold*, which discussed diseases caused by cold, considered an important contribution to the public health because at the time many deaths were attributable to cold, infectious diseases. He also wrote the *Jinkui Yaolue Fanglun* or *Synopsis on Prescriptions of the Golden Chamber* which discussed the origin, symptoms and treatment of skin and various internal diseases. Hua To was a beloved physician who was famous for his use of anesthesia during surgery and his development of the five animal (tiger, deer, bear, bird and monkey) movement exercise to improve circulation and overall health. In acupuncture, the points near the spine were named after him, the huatojiaji points. As the Han dynasty was approaching an end, an important compilation of herbal use that had been passed down from generation to generation since the time of Shen Nong, was published, called the *Shennong Bencaojing* or *Herbal Classic of Shennong*. This book included mineral and animal ingredients in its formulas and was especially utilized and appreciated centuries later in China during the Ming dynasty. Also during the Han dynasty, Zhang Qian opened the Silk Road between the Roman Empire and India, and was consequently considered "the father of the Silk Road." This route expanded not only the trading of goods between western and eastern cultures, but also accelerated the exchange of information ranging from scientific and medical practices to philosophy and religion.

The next three dynasties or Middle Ages were called the Three
Kingdoms Dynasty which lasted from approximately 220 CE to
280 CE, the Jin Dynasty which lasted from 265 CE to 420 CE, and
the Northern and Southern Dynasties which lasted from 420 CE
to 589 CE. During this time span, three important books were
written. Huang Fumi wrote the *Zhenjiu Jiayiying* or *Systemic
Classic of Acupuncture and Moxibustion*. Over 349 acupuncture
points were described and systematized (illustrated by many
acupuncture pathway charts) and the use of moxibustion was just
as comprehensively addressed. Another valuable text was the *Mai
Ching* or *Pulse Classic* written by Wang Shuhe. This book detailed
the significance of 24 different pulses in medical diagnostics.
Ge Hong, an alchemist who formulated "longevity elixirs,"
paradoxically wrote a very practical book entitled *Zhouhou
Beijifang* or *Prescriptions for Emergencies*. In China at this time,
the Xu Xi family rose to preeminence for many generations as
acupuncture and moxibustion experts. Another highlight of this
period was that physicians began teaching medical students more
formally in medical schools, as many were established beginning
in 443 CE.

The science of acupuncture and moxibustion continued to
develop during the Sui Dynasty, which lasted from 581 CE to
618 CE, and during the Tang Dynasty, which lasted from 618 CE
to 917 CE. The Imperial Medical Bureau, which had become
the government agency responsible for medical education,
had four medical specialty departments and one department
of pharmacology; acupuncture was one of those specialty
departments. By 629, government laws enforced certification
examinations in medical schools. A famous doctor, Zhen Quan,
was ordered by the government to revise the medical texts
for acupuncture and moxibustion; he did so, assisted by many
other prominent physicians of the time. Sun Si Miao wrote two
important clinical texts, *Qian Jin Yao Fang* or *Prescriptions
Worth a Thousand Gold for Emergencies* and *Qian Jin Yi Fang*

or *A Supplement to the Prescriptions Worth a Thousand Gold.*
These books distinguished between general diseases, children
and women health concerns, recipes for longevity and, separately,
discussed medical ethics.

During the Five Dynasties, which lasted from 907 CE to 960
CE, the Song Dynasty which lasted from 960 CE to 1279 CE, and
the Yuan Dynasty which lasted from 1271 to 1368 CE, printed
literature describing Chinese medicine and pharmacology was
extensively produced. In 1026, one famous physician, Wang Weiyi,
wrote *Tongren Shuxue Zhen Jia Tujing* or *The Illustrated Manual
on Points for Acupuncture and Moxibustion on a New Bronze
Figure.* In 1027, he designed two life-sized bronze figures with
the meridians and points engraved on the surface for teaching
purposes. Also during this time, anatomical knowledge increased
through the use of dissection.

The Ming Dynasty lasted from 1368 CE to 1644 CE. During this
time, medical theory branched into many different schools of
thought. One group believed that people needed to nourish
their yin energy, while another group believed they needed to
protect their yang energy; one group focused on the treatment of
epidemic diseases (smallpox inoculations were practiced), while
another group felt a return to the classical information without
revision was important; finally, still another group preferred a
moderate healthcare approach by collecting and applying the best
information and practices of all of the other groups. All of this
focus resulted in many changes to acupuncture and moxibustion
during this time, changes like the revision of classical texts
and refinement of clinical techniques. Clinical approaches in
particular changed with the inclusion in patient treatment
of points other than the main meridian points and the use of
warming moxibustion herbs packed in the shape of a stick or
cone. A famous physician, Yang Jizhou, wrote *Zhenjin Dacheng* or
Successful Principles of Acupuncture and Moxibustion. This work
reinforced the principles of the *Nei Jing* and the *Nan Jing.* Herbal
prescriptions became just as important as the actual acupuncture

treatment during this dynasty. Li Shizhen, an innovative doctor and writer, wrote the *Bencao Gangmu* or *Outlines of Roots and Herbs Studies* as an encyclopedia of medicinal ingredients. During this period, plagues began to spread across China; in 1642, in response, a doctor named Wu Youxing published the text *Wenyilun* or *On Pestilence*. He described specific symptoms and treatments for different epidemic diseases.

The Qing Dynasty lasted from 1644 CE until 1911 CE. Led by a physician named Wu Qian, a team of doctors, by imperial order, wrote the *Yizong Jinjuan* or *Golden Mirror of Medicine*. In this book, one chapter, the *Essentials of Acupuncture and Moxibustion,* used rhymed verse with illustrations. While this was considered an important text, Chinese medical doctors had now begun to regard herbal medicine superior to acupuncture and moxibustion. Zhao Xuemin, a physician and famous pharmacist, wrote the *Bencao Gangmu Shiyi* or *Supplement to Compendium of Materia Medica* which listed 921 drugs. He also wrote *Chuanya* or *Treatise on Folk Medicine* which described the teachings of travelling physicians. In 1822, the Imperial Medical College wanted acupuncture and moxibustion removed from its curriculum.

Before, during and after the Opium Wars which lasted from 1839 to 1842 and 1856 to 1860, acupuncture and moxibustion became even less recognized. In fact, Western medicine began to supplant it, as it spread through the country, tethered to the west's growing military power and medical missionary movement. Western missionary hospitals, clinics and medical schools were emerging, and with them, Chinese doctors were introduced first-hand to Western medical practice. Some of these doctors embraced the new knowledge, some resisted this "foreign" intrusion, and still others decided to attempt to integrate both Chinese and Western medicinal thought and practices. In 1892, Zhu Peiwen, a physician and writer, wrote *Huayang Zangxiang Yuezuan* or *A Combining Chinese and Western Anatomy Illustration*, which illustrated organs according to both Chinese and Western concepts and discussed the advantages and disadvantages of each approach. As China moved toward increased medical modernization, an outbreak of the pneumonic plague arrived, known as the great Manchurian plague epidemic of 1910. The Western hygiene and sanitation measures used to combat this outbreak proved very effective and prevented the plague from spreading further throughout China. The Qing Dynasty, and the last dynasty to date, ended in 1911 when the Republic of China was formed.

The Republic of China, or Kuomingtang government, ruled by Sun Yat Sen continued to suppress acupuncture, moxibustion and even herbal medicine while popularizing Western medicine. Based on the experience with the Manchurian plague, public hygiene and Western medicine were preferred for handling the new epidemic diseases such as cholera and diphtheria which were then spreading across China. The Peking Union Medical College, chosen by the Rockefeller foundation in 1915, was a pilot project for establishing a first rate Western medical and teaching center in China. During the May Fourth Movement, in which students in China protested against anything deemed "traditional," modern Western medicine became firmly entrenched as the primary means of curing illness. Even the Central Ministry of Health, established by the government in 1929, preferred Western medicine. Chinese medicine only remained alive by common people offering medical care to the huge population still unattended by Western medicine. These common folk or "barefoot doctors," not only practiced acupuncture, moxibustion and herbal medicine but wrote books, published articles, founded associations and taught correspondence courses. In 1943, the new Kuomingtang or Nationalist government, ruled by Chiang Kaishek, attempted to integrate Chinese and Western medicine by creating a unified "physician's law." This allowed Chinese Medical doctors to qualify for a physician's license and carry equal privileges as Western doctors by meeting one of the following criteria: the physician must have received a diploma from a school of Chinese medicine, passed a government examination or practiced for five years with a "prominent reputation." Another step toward integration occurred in April of 1945, when, at the International Peace Hospital, in the name of Dr. Norman Bethune, an acupuncture clinic was opened. This was the first time that acupuncture and moxibustion were included in a hospital.

In 1949, Chiang Kaishek was forced to retreat to Taiwan by Mao Zedong and the People's Liberation Army. Afterwards, Mao Zedong became chairman of the People's Republic of China. Mao Zedong saw the advantages of expanding the role of the Chinese doctor to meet the needs of the population-at-large; he also shared his foe's vision of uniting Chinese and Western medicine. By 1950, he had established acupuncture in many hospitals. By 1954, the Department of Oriental Medicine was assigned to function under the Ministry of Public Health. However, during the Cultural Revolution, from 1966 to 1976, only the barefoot doctor approach, with its emphasis on treating the common man, was popular, and the expansion of the role of "educated" doctor was not supported. During this time, in 1971, a U.S. reporter named James Reston visited China. Shortly after arriving, he unexpectedly needed an appendectomy. After the surgery, he received acupuncture and moxibustion for pain relief, and he was amazed by the efficacy of the treatment. Reston's reports helped to popularize and promote this alternative approach. Afterwards, as part of the general rapproachment with China engineered by the Nixon administration, an exchange program was instituted that allowed traditional Chinese doctors to come to America to share their medical knowledge and for American doctors to visit China to learn more about this form of treatment. It wasn't until 1980 that the Ministry of Public Health was able to write a national guideline for the development and co-existence of Chinese and Western Medicine in China's healthcare system. Currently, China's healthcare system continues to focus on this integration, and has as its goal universal healthcare with services that are safe, effective, convenient and affordable. One noteworthy discovery that hearkened back to the origins of Chinese medicine occurred as recently as 1973: ancient silk texts, called the Mawangdui texts, were unearthed and found to contain original medical writings, including those contained in the *I Ching* or *Book of Changes* and *Tao Te Ching* or *The Canon of the Tao and its Virtue*.

As we continue to explore the historical development of medicine, we turn to another culture which also incorporated foreign influences into its native approach to medical theory and practice, that of India. Geographically situated between Asia and the European continent, it came to foster its own unique corpus of medical solutions called "Ayurvedic medicine," which can be philosophically thought of as lying between the Chinese and Western traditions we have discussed.

Chinese Medicine Timeline

about 3322 BCE **Fuxi** *wrote* I Ching

2852-2205 BCE *Three Supreme and Five Rulers Dynasty,* **Shen Nong** wrote Pen T'sao *and legendary* **Huangdi** *dialogued with* **Qi Bo**

2100-1600 BCE *Xia Dynasty, nature and man worked together, acupuncture and moxibustion used*

1600-1046 BCE *Shang Dynasty, similar to Xia Dynasty*

1045-256 BCE *Zhou Dynasty,* **Huangdi** *wrote* Nei Jing *and* Nan Jing *written,* **Lao Tzu** *wrote* Tao Te Ching *,* **Zou Yan** *develops Element theory*

221-206 BCE *Qin Dynasty*

206BCE-220CE *Han Dynasty,* **Zhang Zhongjing** *wrote* Shang Han Lun *and* **Hua To** *practiced surgery*

221-280 CE *Three Kingdoms Dynasty*

265-420 CE *Jin Dynasty,* **Wang Shuhe** *wrote* Mai Jing

420-589 CE *Northern and Southern Dynasties, medical schools established*

581-618 CE	*Sui Dynasty, science of acupuncture and moxibustion advanced*
618-907 CE	*Tang Dynasty,* **Sun Si Miao** *wrote* Qian Jin Yao Fang *and* Qian Jin Yi Fang
907-960 CE	*Five Dynasties, extensive printing of Chinese medicine literature*
960-1279 CE	*Song Dynasty, bronze figure engraved with meridians and points*
1271-1368 CE	*Yuan Dynasty, similar to Five Dynasties and Song Dynasty*
1368-1644 CE	*Ming Dynasty, many schools of medical thought, acupuncture and moxibustion refined,* **Li Shizhen** *wrote* Bencao Gangmu, **Wu Youxing** *wrote* Wenyilun
1644-1911 CE	*Qing Dynasty, herbal medicine considered superior to acupuncture and moxibustion,* **Zhao Xuemin** *wrote* Bencao Gangmu Shiyi. *Western medicine introduced.*
1912-1949 CE	*Republic of China, Western medicine preferred and Chinese medicine not supported. Barefoot doctors kept Chinese medicine alive.*
1949-Present	*People's Republic of China, Chinese medicine valued again and the Department of Oriental Medicine assigned to the Ministry of Public Health.*
July 17, 1971	*U.S. reporter,* **James Reston,** *visited China and needed appendectomy, used acupuncture and moxibustion for the pain relief after surgery at the Peking Union Medical College created by the Rockefeller Foundation.*
1973 CE	**Mawangdui** *texts discovered and contained medical writings from the* I Ching *and from the philosophical writings of the* Tao Te Ching.

Part III: History of Ayurvedic Medicine

Similar to the origins of Chinese Medicine, Ayurvedic Medicine has both mythological and historical beginnings. According to myth and religion, the god, Brahma, was in charge of creation while the god, Vishnu, was responsible for preserving creation, and the god, Shiva, had the ability to destroy creation. All of these gods represented one Ultimate God and created the first man, Manu.

Brahma was considered the expansive state of pure existence before light or dark. (Some have drawn a correlation to the modern day scientific theory of an ever-expanding universe.) A grandson to Brahma, avatar to Vishnu, and descendent of Manu named Kapila, passed along this information by describing creation as the journey of awareness evolving into matter. He was a famous philosopher who lived approximately 600 BCE. His philosophies, such as using meditation to calm stress, were similar to the spiritual sage Buddha.

Vishnu supported the universe and maintained its natural and spiritual order or dharma. At times, this order became imbalanced, so Vishnu rescued the good and defeated the evil. One such triumph occurred when Manu was told by a fish that a great flood would destroy all he knew. The fish instructed him to build a large boat and put himself, the animals and plants inside. This fish, actually Vishnu in disguise, also knew that when the flood arrived, the boat would save them all. This story has similarities to the Noah's Ark flood story from the Old Testament of the Bible. Another example, described as the Churning of the Ocean, begins when the bottom of the ocean collected many valuable things. These items needed to be returned, so Vishnu then became a tortoise, named Kurma, and dove courageously to the bottom of the ocean to bring these valuables back. The ocean began swirling and churning as the tortoise tried to swim upward. Gods and demons pushed and pulled on a snake that suddenly surrounded the tortoise, but this pushing and pulling actually

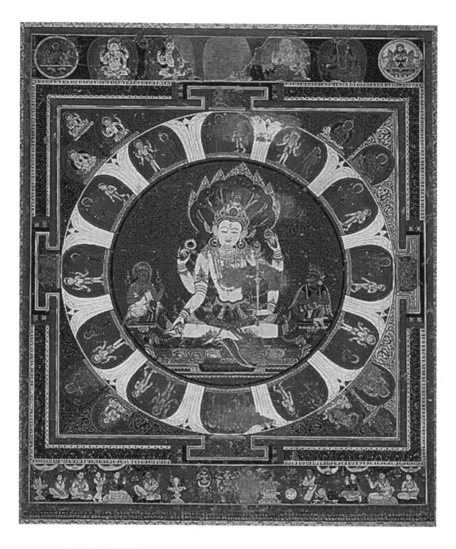

MANDALA OF VISHNU PAINTING, FROM THE NASLI AND ALICE HEERAMANECK COLLECTION,
WIKIMEDIA COMMONS

worked to help restore the valuables to the surface. One important
thing that surfaced was Dhanvantari, the god of Medicine, but
one item that also returned was poison. This endangered all of
mankind. It was important that Shiva now become involved.
Shiva drank the toxin to save humanity and destroy the evil. His
power and spiritual strength removed the suffering of the world.

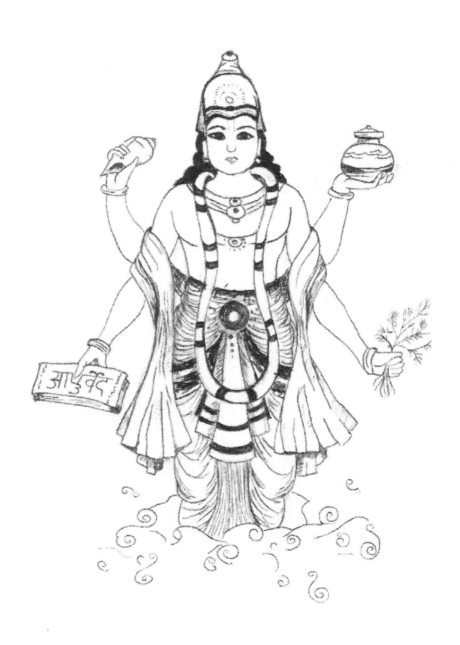

DHANVANTARI, GOD OF MEDICINE, ILLUSTRATED BY SARAH NICITA

Brahma, Vishnu and Shiva, along with their respective creative, preservative and destructive powers, were destined to maintain a balance in the universe.

Dhanvantari, who was returned to the surface in this myth, was also a grandson of Brahma and the founder of Ayurveda or the "science of life" medicine. He is believed to have become wise in the ways of optimal health by listening to the gods during meditation. Afterwards, he in turn taught this information to mortal sages. It is at this time that something resembling a true historical record of Ayurvedic medicine begins.

In approximately 8000 BCE, Atreya, a great Ayurvedic master, wrote the oldest medical book in the world, the *Atreya Samhita*. It had many chapters and discussed the eight main branches of Ayurveda: internal medicine, surgery, fertility, pediatrics, psychiatry, toxicology, anti-aging and ears, eyes and nose.

Estimated at 3000 to 2000 BCE, a famous sage and avatar to Vishnu, Bhagavan Sri VedaVyasa, codified Ayurvedic medical and spiritual information into books or *Vedas*. The oldest of these texts was the *Rig Veda*. It contained information regarding disease and treatment options such as surgery (including organ transplants), herbs with great curative properties, yoga, essential oils, and recommended food adjustments and lifestyle changes. Another of these famous Vedas was the *Sama Veda*. It contained holy hymns. A companion veda was the *Yajur Veda*, primarily recording religious rituals. For example, mantras containing particular sounds, words or songs were documented, to be repeated during meditation. Lastly, the *Atharva Veda* was also written at this time, containing specific information about each of the eight main areas of focus in Ayurveda originally treated in the *Atreya Samhita*.

Around 1500 to 1000 BCE, Ayurvedic medicine followed a similar developmental path as Western and Chinese medicine by evolving from a religious discipline into a medical system with many specializations. In particular, two schools of medicine were founded: Atreya, as a school for physicians and Dhanvantari, as a school for surgeons. Two significant books, the *Charaka Samhita* and the *Susruta Samhita*, were written during this time. The *Charaka Samhita* was authored by the physician Charaka, considered to be "the father of Ayurvedic medicine." Digestion, immunity and metabolism were discussed in this internal medicine textbook. The *Susruta Samhita* was written by the physician Susruta, named "the father of Ayurvedic surgery." Amputation, brain and cosmetic surgery are described in this equally important medical textbook. Marma points are noted: these points on the body are similar to acupuncture points. Around 500 CE, these two texts were followed by a third, called the *Ashtanga Hridaya Samhita*. Together, these three medical texts became known as the "Senior Triad." The next important written contribution to the development of Ayurveda was that of the physician Vhagbhatta, who wrote the *Ashtanga Hridaya Samhita*. This compilation of medical material combined internal medicine and surgical information into one book. These influential manuals were "published" and to some degree "circulated" during the Golden Age of India, approximately 1000 BCE to 800 CE. The medical information they contained became popular not just with native Indians, but also with the Egyptians, Greeks, Romans, Chinese, Tibetans, Persians and Arabs who travelled to India to glean the secrets of Ayurvedic medical knowledge. After their studies were completed, they brought back these valuable insights to their own cultures.

As part of this information migration, during the Middle Ages, from approximately 1000 CE to 1200 CE, the physicians Rhazes and Avicenna translated much of this Ayurvedic medical wisdom into Arabic. Unfortunately, the spread of Ayurvedic medicine began to decline as the Muslims invaded India. Medical universities and libraries were burned. The Muslims practiced "Unani Tibb" medicine exclusively at that time, a combination of Greek and Islamic medicine, based on work dating as far back as Hippocrates and Galen, further developed by others, most notably Avicenna. This medical approach was also favored in Europe. Hindus, however, despite the growing Muslim influence, continued to use their ancient Ayurveda. One important medical book that was written in approximately 1100 CE, by Madhava Charya, was called the *Madhava Nidanam*. This text described and classified diseases about children, women, toxicology, and the ear, nose and throat. It is the first of three significant works that would come to make up the "Junior Triad" of Ayurvedic medicine.

The second member of the Junior Triad was the *Sharangdhara Samhita* written by Acharya Sharangdhara in approximately 1300 CE. This book included information about new syndromes, their treatments, herbal and pharmacological formulas and pulse diagnosis. The final part of the Junior Triad reference was a text called the *Bhava Prakasha,* authored by Bhava Mishra around 1500 CE. This valuable book reorganized the two earlier works and discussed many medicinal characteristics of food, plants and minerals. It is also during this time that Paracelsus, the great Swiss Renaissance physician, is greatly influenced by the growing corpus of Ayurvedic medical knowledge.

When Mughal Emperor Akbar ruled India during the mid-1500's, Ayurveda again began to flourish. Akbar was open-minded and encouraged Western and Indian physicians to exchange information. For example, Garcia D'Orta, a Portuguese doctor and naturalist, printed an Indian medical book called *Conversations on the Medical Simples and Drugs of India* in 1563. He collected information about disease case studies and plant properties from many local physicians as part of his extensive research for this work.

Unfortunately, in the 1600's, feuding began between the Portuguese and Indians. One consequence was that the Portuguese outlawed Hindu physicians. In addition, the British, in the form of the British East India Company, began arriving at the beginning of the 1600's, and establishing a colonial empire across most of India. However, at the end of the 1600's, a more positive exchange occurred when the Dutch East India Company showed great interest in the local Indian plants and flowers. In particular, Hendrik van Rheede, a Dutch colonial governor and naturalist, prepared, with help from a small army of physicians and botanists, the comprehensive *Hortus Malabaricus,* a 12 volume set that described approximately eight hundred Indian plants and their medicinal properties. These volumes were published in Amsterdam between the years of 1686 and 1703.

By 1833, the British East India Company had banned all Ayurvedic medical institutions and opened the first Western medical university in Calcutta. During this time, as was the case in China, Ayurvedic medicine was kept alive only in the rural areas where people either could not afford Western medicine, or were geographically dispersed from the larger urban areas where it was available. Any Ayurveda training was received from a private college or taught by families secretly sharing medical information with each other. By 1858, the East India Company disbanded and India was ruled under the British crown. The *British Pharmacopoeia* became widely used, a standardized compilation of Western drugs. Its popularity helped to further decrease the medicinal use of Ayurveda plants, flowers and herbs.

However by 1920, Indian nationalism was increasing under the leadership of Ghandi and with it, the more traditional aspects of Indian culture, including Ayurveda, were being rediscovered. In fact, when India received its independence from the British in 1947, Ayurvedic medical schools were reopened. Today, there are many colleges in India practicing and teaching Ayurveda. Ayurvedic doctors are working with Western doctors in hospitals to provide the best complementary medical care. As one sign of the growth and popularity of this approach, The All-India Ayurveda Congress now counts itself as the largest medical organization in the world.

There are many similar patterns that can be drawn from a comparison of the historical development of these three major schools of Western, Chinese and Ayurvedic medicine. One not mentioned so far is that they share similar "do no harm" and "life is sacred" philosophies despite all of the significant cultural contexts, different treatment protocols and varying diagnostic approaches. Their native development has been closely intertwined with political and cultural events, a pattern that continues to this day. And just as the evolution of each of these traditions has been characterized by a great deal of synthesis of "foreign" influences, so too are we today at a juncture that allows us to embrace an approach that incorporates the best practices across all three models into one unified, holistic, multi-cultural, patient-based model. The following chapters will build upon these historical foundations to compare Western, Chinese and Ayurvedic theories and practices as a prelude to the creation of just such a new model.

Ayurvedic Medicine Timeline

Vedic Age

8000 BCE	**Atreya Samhita**
3500 BCE	**VedaVyasa** *wrote Ayurveda information in* Vedas
3000 BCE	Rig Veda, Sama Veda, Yajur Veda
2000 BCE	Atharva Veda
1500 BCE	*two schools formed- the Dhanvantari school taught Ayurveda and the Atreya school taught surgery*

Golden Age

1000 BCE	*two books of Senior Triad are written- the* Charaka Samhita *and the* Susruta Samhita
500 CE	*third Senior Triad book written-* Ashtanga Hridaya Samhita; *Ayurveda spreads globally*

Middle Ages

1000-1200 CE	*Muslim invasion, Ayurveda began to decline*
1100 CE	*first of Junior Triad books written- the* Madhava Nidanam
1300 CE	*second of Junior Triad books written- the* Sharangdhara Samhita
1500 CE	*third of Junior Triad books written-* Bhava Prakasha
Mid- 1500's	**Mughal Emperor Akbar** *ruled, Indian and Western physicians exchange information*
1563	**Garcia D'Orta** *wrote* Conversations on the Medical Simples and Drugs of India

British Imperialism Age

1600's	*East India Company began to conquer India*
1686-1703	**Hendrik van Rheede** *compiles* Hortus Malabaricus
1833	*East India Company banned all Ayurveda institutions*
1858	*East India Company dissolved and India ruled under British crown,* British Pharmacopoeia *published*
1920	**Ghandi** *increased Indian nationalism support*

Modern Age

1947	*Indian independence, Ayurvedic medical schools reopened*
Current	**All-India Ayurveda Congress,** *largest medical organization in the world*

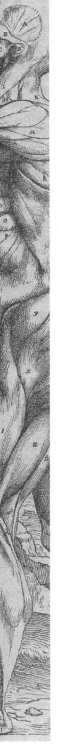

Chapter Two:
Anatomical and Physiological Theory and Philosophy, Diagnosis and Treatment Principles of Western, Chinese and Ayurvedic Medicine

"A clash of doctrine is not a disaster, it is an opportunity."
-ALFRED NORTH WHITEHEAD

This chapter will provide an overview of the similarities and differences between Western, Chinese and Ayurvedic medicine regarding anatomy, physiology, diagnosis of diseases and treatment protocols.

Western medicine offers a scientific, linear approach to describing the human body and uses atoms, molecules, cells, genes, tissues, organs and systems to explain its anatomy and physiology. Atoms are the small particles that build and make matter. When two or more atoms unite, a molecule is formed. These molecules usually have two or more different atoms. An example is the water molecule. This molecule contains one atom of oxygen and two atoms of hydrogen.

The cell is the basic unit of every living animal or plant. Cells contain water, protein, sugar, acids, fats, and various minerals. The cell has a control center or nucleus which contains hereditary or genetic material called chromosomes. Inside the chromosome are thousands of genes. The gene is composed of DNA or deoxyribonucleic acid. These DNA molecules decide human inherited characteristics such as green eyes.

Tissues are a group of similar cells working together to do specialized work. For example, the outside of the body and the inner surface of internal body organs like the stomach are lined with epithelial tissue. Throughout the body, messages or impulses are transmitted by nerve tissue. Except for the brain and the spinal cord, nerve tissue is supported by connective tissue. Connective tissue is either soft in the form of fat, fibrous like tendons or ligaments, or hard as cartilage or bone. Muscle tissue's purpose is to allow the body to move. Muscle tissue found in the arms or legs can contract or extend when it is called on to do so, and is therefore considered voluntary, while muscle tissue found in the heart or digestive systems is considered involuntary because there is no conscious control over its movement.

Organs are composed of two or more of the above mentioned tissues- epithelial, nerve, connective or muscle. Here is a list of the major organs and some of their functions:

Heart- *governs blood circulation, releases deoxygenated blood for oxygen-rich blood.*

Pericardium- *surrounds and protects the heart.*

Lung- *allows oxygen to be inhaled and carbon dioxide exhaled, while gases are exchanged at the cellular level.*

Spleen- *stores blood and removes pathogens from the blood, activates lymphocytes, and destroys old red blood cells.*

Pancreas- *produces enzymes to digest food and secretes insulin.*

Stomach- *is characterized by involuntary movement, and contains hydrochloric acid and enzymes that break down food, which it then mixes with mucus to become chyme. The chyme is received by the small intestine for further digestion and absorption into the bloodstream.*

Liver- *detoxifies blood, keeps blood glucose at a normal level, and produces bile which contains cholesterol, bile acids and bilirubin. Bilirubin is a released when old red blood cells are destroyed.*

Gall Bladder- *stores and concentrates bile.*

Small Intestine- *helps food absorption after receiving food from the stomach, bile from the liver and gall bladder and pancreatic juice from the pancreas.*

Large Intestine- *absorbs water from waste products then uses involuntary movement or peristalsis to push waste products from the body.*

Kidney- *removes urea, maintains the proper balance of water,salts and acids in body fluids, and produces hormones such as rennin to control blood pressure and erythropoietin to regulate red blood cell production.*

Urinary Bladder- *stores urine.*

Systems are groups of organs working together to perform complicated and intricate functions. Here is a list of our human body's ten systems:

Digestive- *mouth, throat, esophagus, stomach, intestines, liver, gall bladder, pancreas*

Urinary- *kidneys, ureters, urinary bladder, urethra*

Respiratory- *nose, pharynx, larynx, trachea, bronchial tubes, lungs*

Reproductive- *females have ovaries, fallopian tubes, uterus, vagina, and mammary glands and males have testes with tubes, urethra, penis and a prostate gland*

Endocrine- *thyroid gland, pituitary gland, sex glands- ovaries and testes, adrenal glands, pancreas, parathyroid glands, pineal gland, thymus gland*

Nervous- *brain, spinal cord, nerves and collections of nerves*

Circulatory- *heart, blood vessels, lymphatic vessels and nodes, spleen, thymus gland*

Muscular- *muscles*

Skeletal- *bones and joints*

Skin and sense organs- *skin, hair, nails, sweat glands and oil glands, eyes, ears, nose, and tongue*

Symptoms are studied at these levels to understand the cause of the illness or problem. To aid in the diagnosis, questions are asked about the nature of the symptoms, a family history is required and an exam of the problem area is explored by palpation or technological equipment such as an X-ray, ultrasound or MRI. The treatment focuses on controlling or eliminating the unwanted disease or ailment to restore health and includes drug therapy, surgery, physical therapy, massage and/or nutrition advice.

Let's now take a look at Chinese medicine's healthcare approach. According to the *Su Wen* of the *Nei Jing*, "Waiting to treat illness after they manifest is like waiting to dig a well after one is thirsty." Chinese medicine is a holistic, integrative medicine that considers illnesses and harmony in the human body as a combination of physical, emotional, mental, spiritual and environmental factors. Disease is due to a disturbance in one of these areas. To determine the imbalance, Chinese medicinal philosophy uses combinations of the Eight Principles (yin/yang, exterior/ interior, excess/deficiency, hot/cold), the Seven Emotions (joy, anger, sadness, worry, grief, fear, fright), the Six Environmental Influences (wind, cold, summer heat, dampness, dryness, fire), and the Five Elements (wood, fire, earth, metal, water) along with qi, blood, body fluids and organ analysis to describe its diagnosis methodology.

With regard to the Eight Principles, yin and yang are terms referring to the two aspects of the universe which are opposite yet completely dependent upon one another. Some examples are night and day, dark and light, cold and hot, quiet and active, down and up, front and back, foot and head, earth and heaven and the symbols of a phoenix and a dragon. Not only are yin and yang opposing forces that are interdependent, yin and yang consume and support, transform, and continually change and control each other. If yin lessens, then yang will increase and support the condition. If yin lessens to an extreme, then the condition will become yang. For example, if a severe yin cold exists, a severe yang heat will arise.

As previously mentioned, the Seven Emotions are joy, anger, sadness, worry, grief, fear and fright. These emotions are associated with certain organs. Joy goes with the heart and anger with the liver, sadness is associated with the lung and worry with the spleen, and fear or fright is connected with the kidney. If someone worries too much, the spleen can be injured; if someone has excess anger, the liver can become damaged.

As for the Six Environmental Factors - wind, cold, summer heat, dampness, dryness and fire – all can cause seasonal diseases. For example, colds occur mostly in the winter because the temperature is colder than the rest of the year and more wind or dampness is prevalent. In fact, "wind can be the cause of 100 different diseases," according to the *Su Wen*. The wind pushes the pathogen into the body through the skin, mouth or nose. These Eight Principles, Seven Emotions and Six Environmental Factors are important to consider when assessing the cause of an imbalance in the human body, but the Five Element Theory is also very helpful in understanding the origin of an illness.

The Five Elements Theory maintains that all things in the universe correlate to wood, fire, earth, metal and water, and are always changing and moving. The wood grows and flourishes, the fire is hot and flares up, the earth gives birth to all things, the metal descends and clears, and the water is cold and flows downward. This theory was first described by the philosopher Zou Yin. These elements, phases or energies transform into one another in a cyclical, orderly manner. The balance is sustained through cycles of creation and destruction of these elements or phases.

The creation or generating cycle begins with the wood element. It represents birth and beginnings. For example, rubbing two pieces of wood together creates fire, the firewood incinerates into ashes, and the ashes become the earth. The earth produces metal ores which melt into liquid. This liquid or water sprouts wood. This cycle is repeated over and over again.

The destructive or controlling cycle starts with the example of water putting out fire. The fire then melts down the metal. The metal is shaped into an axe that cuts apart the wood. The wood roots permeate the earth and the earth holds the water. This cycle is also repeated over and over again.

With the human body, each element has organ connections.

Wood corresponds to the liver and gall bladder, fire to the heart and small intestine, earth to the spleen and stomach, metal to the lung and large intestine and water to the kidney and urinary bladder. Health occurs when an organ is supported, controlled and receiving nourishment from its proper corresponding elements.

Also needed for vitality are the basic substances of the human body- qi, blood and body fluids. Qi is the life force that permeates the human body. Its main functions are to promote growth and circulation of blood and fluid in the body, maintain normal body temperature, defend the body from pathogens, control and transform metabolic products and body substances, and help ingested food to nourish the body.

Blood is a red fluid that circulates throughout the body in vessels. The blood nourishes and moistens all the organs and tissues. Sufficient blood keeps bones and tendons strong, joints moving smoothly, the mind keen and alert and the spirit soaring with vigor.

Besides blood, body fluids that are thick and heavy or thin and watery, such as saliva, gastric or intestinal juices, joint cavity substances, urine, sweat, nasal discharge and tears, also nourish and moisten the body. All three basic substances - qi, blood and body fluids - work together. Qi is the yang and provides movement and warmth, while blood and the other body fluids, represent the yin and provide nourishment and moisture for the organs of the body.

The organs of the body have both physiological functions and energetic significance. The organs are classified into zang or fu types. Zang organs are the solid organs that store important substances such as qi, blood and body fluids. They consist of the heart, pericardium, lung, spleen, liver and kidney. Fu organs are the hollow organs that receive and digest food or transport waste. They consist of the gall bladder, stomach, small intestine, large intestine, urinary bladder and san jiao. There are even "extraordinary" fu organs- the brain, marrow, bones, vessels, gall bladder and uterus. These organs function like a zang organ but have the hollow shape of a fu organ. For example, the gall bladder stores bile, but does not receive water or food, and has a hollow shape, so it is considered an extraordinary organ.

The organ energy pathways are called meridians. These pathways connect the organs, the upper and lower limbs, the internal and external parts of the body and regulate bodily functions. These meridians contain qi.

Here is a description of the major organs in Chinese medicine and some of their functions:

The Zang or yin organs

Heart- *governs and pushes blood, controls blood vessels, manifest in skin color, (especially the face), houses mental and spiritual activity, consciousness, memory, thinking and sleeping, open into the tongue and is associated with the emotion of joy.*

Pericardium- *governs blood, protects the heart and houses the mind.*

Lung- *governs qi and respiration, controls dispersing and descending, regulates water passages, controls skin and hair, opens into the nose and is associated with the emotion of sadness or grief.*

Spleen- *governs the transformation and transportation of food into qi and blood, controls blood by keeping blood in the vessels, nourishes muscles and the four limbs, manifests on the lips, and is associated with the emotion of worry.*

Liver- *stores blood, promotes smooth flow of qi, controls tendons, manifests in the nails, opens into the eyes and is* *associated with the emotions of anger.*

Kidney- *stores essence, governs birth, growth, reproduction and development, controls bones, produces marrow, governs water metabolism, controls receiving qi, manifests in the hair, opens into the ears, houses willpower and is associated with the emotion of fear or fright.*

The Fu or yang organs

Stomach- *controls rotting and ripening of food, transportation of food essences and the descending of qi.*

Gall Bladder- *stores and excretes bile, helps liver with flow of qi, and controls decision- making.*

Small Intestine- *Receives and further digests food from the stomach, clears the turbid and absorbs essential nutrients; afterwards sends food to the large intestine and water to the urinary bladder.*

Large Intestine- *receives food from small intestine, absorbs its fluid content and then excretes waste.*

Urinary Bladder- *stores urine.*

San Jiao- *is unique to Chinese medicine's anatomy and physiology. The San Jiao has three sections: upper, middle and lower. The upper jiao disperses the essential qi of food and water to the whole body. The middle jiao digests, absorbs and transforms nutrients in food. The lower jiao separates the clear from the turbid and gets rid of unwanted fluids and wastes from the body.*

Since the vessels, bones, marrow and gall bladder have already been mentioned, only the brain and uterus will be noted next as extraordinary organs.

Two Extraordinary organs

Brain- *is also called "the sea of marrow," and is the organ of spirit, consciousness and thinking.*

Uterus- *controls menstruation and nourishes the fetus.*

To discern the pattern of disharmony, a Chinese medicine doctor asks questions about the patient's past, present and family health history, looks at the tongue, checks wrist pulses in a very specific way, notices odors, and palpates the topography of meridians and possibly the abdomen.

Once the imbalance is determined, acupuncture, herbs, moxibustion, cupping, nutrition guidance or specialized tai chi or qi gong exercises are then prescribed to naturally restore the order of health. Acupuncture is the insertion of fine needles into specific points along the body. Moxibustion is an herbal substance that is heated and held above or placed directly on top of specific points along the body. Cupping is the process of heating glass cups or pumping plastic air cups and then placing them on the skin or sliding the glass cups along the skin.

Having surveyed the anatomical and physiological approaches of both Western and Chinese medicine, let's now review the Ayruvedic view of these systems. Ayurveda uses Western's extensive knowledge of anatomy and its linear understanding of disease progression but combines this with a holistic, integrative approach to healthcare that in some ways parallels Chinese medicine. One of these parallels is the way that Ayurvedic medicine attunes itself with the laws of nature and believes any physical, mental or spiritual imbalance can also cause illness. According to Ayurveda philosophy, nature has three important qualities or *gunas*, that exist everywhere and are necessary for creation. These gunas are *sattva*, *rajas* and *tamas*. Sattva creates balance and lightness, rajas produces movement and activity and tamas brings stillness and heaviness.

The basic Ayurvedic philosophy also utilizes the five great elements (space, air, fire, water, earth) and identifies the three *doshas,* known as *pitta, kapha* and *vata,* to determine your *pakruti,* or inherent constitution or personality, to form the basis of diagnosis and treatment of disease. The seven tissues (plasma, blood, muscle, fat, bone, nerve and reproductive), the three wastes, digestive fire, toxicity symptoms and organ or system ailments are also analyzed.

The five elements have a hierarchical structure and begin with ether. Ether, or *akasha,* creates air. Air, or *vayu,* is found in space and can create heat which eventually becomes fire. Fire, or *tejas,* then melts into water, and water, or *apas,* hardens and becomes earth, or *pruthivi.* These elements have physiological and emotional representations. Ether or space is found everywhere in the body. For example, ether surrounds joints, arteries, the respiratory system, gastrointestinal tract, even the cells themselves. The balanced emotion is feeling peaceful and the imbalanced emotion is fear. Air is mostly utilized by the lung and large intestine, governs cellular movement and represents the positive emotion joy or the negative emotion sadness. Fire helps with the digestion, absorption and the changing of food into energy, governs body temperature, fuels intelligence and the balanced emotion is associated with appreciation and the imbalanced emotion with anger. Water is the bodily liquid found in plasma, blood, sweat, saliva, urine and cytoplasm and the positive emotion is connected with compassion and the negative emotion is connected with greed. Earth is the physical substance seen in bones, cartilage, tendons, nails and provides cellular structure and support; the balanced emotion is feeling centered while the imbalanced emotion is feeling depressed.

The five elements are seen in the three doshas- vata, pitta, and kapha. For example, space and air create vata, fire and water form pitta, and water and earth appear in kapha. The five elements govern the structure of the human body while the three doshas regulate the body's functions.

Vata is associated with the brain, lungs, heart, bones, bone marrow and nervous system. It is responsible for all bodily movement and activity. The qualities of vata are dry, cold, light, irregular, moving and rough.

Pitta is associated with the liver, small intestine, spleen, brain, blood, eyes and skin and endocrine systems. It is responsible for digestion and metabolism. The qualities of pitta are oily, hot, light, intense, odorous and liquid.

Kapha is associated with the stomach, brain, mouth, joints and the lymph system. It is responsible for the lubrication of the body. The qualities of kapha are oily, cold, heavy, stable, dense and smooth.

To help the body structure exist and function, the seven tissues are necessary. These tissues are plasma or *rasa*, blood or *rakta*, muscle or *mamasa*, fat or *meda*, bone or *asthi*, nerve and blood marrow or *majja*, and reproductive or *shukra* for male and *artava* for female. Plasma supports the lymphatic system, blood is the substance of the circulatory system, muscle allows for body movement, fat maintains the body temperature, bones compose the skeletal system, nerves send messages throughout the body, the bone marrow supports the bones and the reproductive tissues create new bodies. When the body has healthy tissues a special substance, called *ojas*, is created and keeps the immune system strong. The body prefers ojas to *ama*, otherwise known as body toxins. These toxins need to be released from the three bodily wastes or *malas*- sweat, feces and urine. In addition, the digestive fire, or *agni*, that exists throughout the body needs to be functioning at its best to keep the body in balance.

The anatomy and physiology of the human body in Ayurvedic

medicine is similar to Western medicine. (Please refer to Western medicine's anatomy and physiology previously described in this chapter for details.) The organs and systems are definitely important to discuss when trying to identify any imbalances in the body. The emotional and energetic information of the body, however, is equally significant. Ayurvedic medicine has energy points called *marmas* and energy centers called *chakras*. Marma points are specific body spots that contain the life force or *prana*. These points also regulate the harmony of the body, mind, emotions and soul. Even during surgery, it is recommended that marma points are avoided so as not to deplete the life force in the body. The energy from the marma points connect to the chakras. Chakras are seven energy centers located along the base of the spine to the top of the head. The first chakra, or *muladhara*, is located at the base of the spine and focuses on helping a person feeling grounded and making certain that their basic survival needs are met. The second chakra, or *svadhisthana*, is located at the area of the reproductive organs and helps to develop positive self-esteem and a healthy sex drive. The third chakra, or *manipura*, is located at the level of the solar plexus and focuses on facilitating the development of a person's power and ambition. The fourth chakra, or *anahata*, is located at the heart and is responsible for cultivating compassion and love in a person. The fifth chakra, or *vishuddhi*, is located at the throat and helps develop clear communication and self-expression in a person. The sixth chakra, or *ajna,* is located between the eyebrows and focuses on aiding in the growth of a person's intuitive abilities. The seventh chakra, or *sahasrara,* is located on the top of the head and is responsible for the movement toward obtaining enlightenment and experiencing bliss.

During a treatment, Ayurveda inquires about the past, present and family history, checks the tongue and palpates the pulses in a specific way, looks at the eyes and nails and listens to the heart, lungs and intestines. Identifying the elemental and dosha imbalances, discussing the tissue concerns, the metabolic wastes and digestive fire function, and reviewing any organ or system ailment is part of the intake during an appointment.

To treat illness or imbalances, Ayurveda's "science of life" medicine combines massage, surgery, herbal medicine, mental, emotional and lifestyle counselling, meditation, yoga and nutrition. For example, massage therapies used in this therapeutic manner aim to physically cleanse or detoxify the body as well as calm, nourish or rejuvenate the body and mind; they are called *panchakarma*.

All three healthcare modalities use observation and questioning the patient as diagnostic tools. Western medicine doctors look at the tongue when symptoms, like a sore throat, indicate that this is necessary, and feel the wrist pulse to count the number of beats per minute to check on heart health; Chinese and Ayurvedic medicine practitioners look at the tongue and feel the wrist pulse to obtain energetic information in order to understand the cause of the imbalance in the body. Physical, mental and emotional symptoms are of primary concern when seeing a Western medical doctor, while a Chinese or Ayurvedic practitioner not only considers those symptoms, but also incorporates and evaluate energetic, environmental and spiritual issues into the formulation of a diagnosis and treatment plan. Western medicine does not acknowledge a life force in the body while both Chinese and Ayurvedic medicine, believe wholeheartedly that a life force exists and is important to healthy somatic function and vitality. Chinese medicine calls this life energy qi and Ayurvedic medicine refers to this life force as prana. Both Chinese and Ayurvedic medicine attune themselves to the laws of nature even though they have different philosophies for describing how the body operates. Ayurveda has similar anatomy, physiology and disease progression as Western medicine, while Chinese medicine includes energetic information in its anatomy and physiology understanding and describes disease progression in patterns. All three healthcare modalities consider how the body and mind affect each other, but it is only Chinese and Ayurvedic medicine that hold that spiritual disconnect can cause illness. Regarding treatment, surgery is used in Western and Ayurvedic medicine while acupuncture, moxibustion and cupping are the preferred courses of treatment in Chinese medicine. Drugs are primarily promoted in Western medicine while herbal preparations are the main recommendations in Chinese and Ayurvedic medicine. The next chapter will explore Western medicine's drug therapy along with Chinese and Ayurveda's herbal medicine approach. Lifestyle and nutrition counseling, exercise and meditative prayer are important to all three healthcare approaches.

In today's world, using allopathic or natural medicine is an important way to restore health. One way to record personally significant health information is to keep a medical history diary. If you visit the **vitalityfusion.com** website, you can print your own copy of the following medical history form, to keep track of your health. (For future updates, make copies of the website form before completing.) Also include with this form any lab results or X-rays. Maintaining a current and complete personal medical history can be the first step in becoming your own best health advocate.

Medical health history form

The following will be your personal health record. Please keep other medical records such as blood tests or X-rays with this diary to help organize your history. Make copies of this blank form to update information as needed.

Today's Date:

List current medical doctors and other health practitioners below:

Name _____
Address _____
Phone _____

Name _____
Address _____
Phone _____

Name _____
Address _____
Phone _____

Family History
Please list all immediate family members who have had a history of arthritis, asthma, cancer, diabetes, heart disease such as high blood pressure or stroke, hepatitis, low blood sugar, kidney disease, mental illness or tuberculosis.

Family Member   Disease

_____   _____
_____   _____
_____   _____

Personal History
Weight _____
Height _____
Blood Pressure _____
Blood Type_____

Immunization Records:
Tetanus _____
Whooping Cough _____
Diphtheria_____
Polio_____
Chicken Pox _____
Measles _____
Mumps _____

Surgery History:
Date   Type

_____   _____
_____   _____
_____   _____
_____   _____

List any allergies

_____
_____
_____
_____

Do you smoke?_____
Do you drink alcohol? _____
What are your current health concerns or goals?

_____
_____
_____
_____
_____

Body Inquiry

On a scale of one through ten, where one indicates feeling great without disease and ten signifies excruciating pain and dysfunction, answer the following questions. Include other comments in the qualitative area to complete your description. For example, with the first question, describe your energy level? You can answer by circling the number five, then write, "I have a medium amount of energy." Or for the skin texture question, you can circle number eight, then write, "I have acne and rashes on my face and chest."

Describe:	Quantitative	Qualitative
Your energy level?	1 2 3 4 5 6 7 8 9 10	
Your sleeping pattern?	1 2 3 4 5 6 7 8 9 10	
Your skin texture?	1 2 3 4 5 6 7 8 9 10	
Any headaches?	1 2 3 4 5 6 7 8 9 10	
Any neck pain?	1 2 3 4 5 6 7 8 9 10	
Any backaches?	1 2 3 4 5 6 7 8 9 10	
Any hip pain?	1 2 3 4 5 6 7 8 9 10	
Any knee pain?	1 2 3 4 5 6 7 8 9 10	
Any vision problems?	1 2 3 4 5 6 7 8 9 10	
Any hearing problems?	1 2 3 4 5 6 7 8 9 10	

Describe:	Quantitative	Qualitative
Any cold hands or feet?	1 2 3 4 5 6 7 8 9 10	
Any belching?	1 2 3 4 5 6 7 8 9 10	
Any bad breath?	1 2 3 4 5 6 7 8 9 10	
Any constipation?	1 2 3 4 5 6 7 8 9 10	
Any diarrhea?	1 2 3 4 5 6 7 8 9 10	
Any lack of appetite?	1 2 3 4 5 6 7 8 9 10	
Any food cravings?	1 2 3 4 5 6 7 8 9 10	
Any sinus congestion?	1 2 3 4 5 6 7 8 9 10	
Any breathing difficulty?	1 2 3 4 5 6 7 8 9 10	
Any thirst?	1 2 3 4 5 6 7 8 9 10	
Any sweating?	1 2 3 4 5 6 7 8 9 10	
Any bloating?	1 2 3 4 5 6 7 8 9 10	
Any abdominal pain?	1 2 3 4 5 6 7 8 9 10	
Any colds or flus?	1 2 3 4 5 6 7 8 9 10	
Any chest pain?	1 2 3 4 5 6 7 8 9 10	

The following diagrams will help you illustrate the health of your body. Write in where it hurts or mark the body regions that seem to be out of balance. For example, if you have frequent headaches, write the word headache across the forehead of this diagram. Decide if the face is smiling or looking frustrated. Include comments where your body is feeling strong. For example, if your skin is clear and smooth, you can draw a line to the body and write great-looking skin.

Female chart

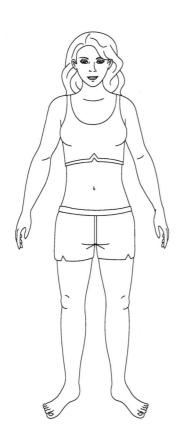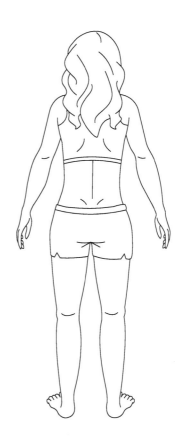

Male chart

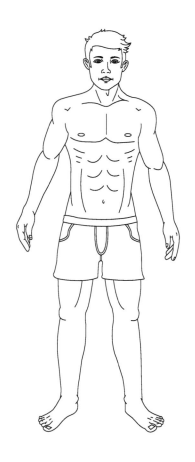 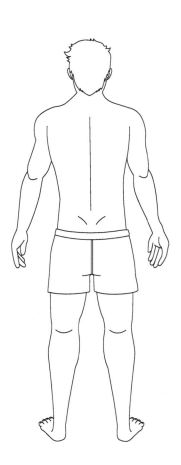

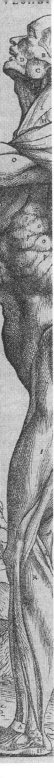

Chapter Three:
Herbal Medicine and
Pharmaceuticals

*"Herbs (medicines), while descending down from heaven to
earth proclaimed those who eat us, are never destroyed."*

-YAJUR VEDA

This chapter will discuss some basic information about Western
herbal medicine and pharmaceuticals as well as Chinese and
Ayurvedic herbal medicine. This type of medicine can cure and
eliminate dysfunction and disease, if the prescription given is
accurately formulated and properly dosed. Let's first take a look
at how herbal medicine and pharmaceuticals were used in the
West to create this restorative healing.

Herbs, defined as broadly as possible, can come from
fruits, flowers, seeds, leaves, bark, stems, rhizomes, roots,
animals, shells or minerals. As mentioned in Chapter One,
herbal medicine has been around since prehistoric times.
Approximately 60,000 years ago, herbal use was evident at a
Neanderthal burial site near Iraq. The *Ebers Papyrus* (previously
mentioned in Chapter One) contained herbal prescriptions.
Around 400 BCE, Hippocrates wrote about medicinal plants

and their curative effects. In 70 CE, Dioscorides, a physician and herbalist, published *De Materia Medica,* or *On Medicinal Substances*, consisting of five volumes. This highly regarded medical reference gave the plant name with an illustration, described the properties, actions and uses of the herbal medicine and noted side effects, dosage and storage instructions. In the 1500's, Paracelsus, a famous physician who was considered "the father of toxicology," researched and experimented with substances to understand their action and interaction with each other. He discovered, paradoxically, that toxic substances used in a small dose may be beneficial, while benign substances over-consumed can be lethal. At the beginning of the 1800's, Francois Magendie, a French physiologist who was considered "the father of experimental pharmacology," isolated emetine from ipecac and researched the effects of drugs on the body. Among his discoveries was the fact that chemical substances were absorbed through the bloodstream and the skin, and not the lymph system.

Pharmacology is the study of drugs. Drugs are biological materials such as plants or animals or chemicals that are usually produced synthetically, while still retaining their chemically similarity to the original natural substance. They are developed and manufactured to restore health and/or fight disease. For example, digitalis comes from the foxglove plant, penicillin comes from mold and prednisone comes from laboratory-synthesized chemicals.

There are different areas of pharmacological study. Medicinal chemistry looks at the chemical structure and biological effects of a new drug while pharmacodynamics is the study of drug effects on the body with regard to its absorption, metabolism and excretion. Pharmacokinetics describes the appearance and disappearance of the drug in the body as a mathematical measurement while molecular pharmacology studies how a drug interacts at the subcellular level, on such structures as RNA, DNA or enzymes. Chemotherapy is the study of drugs that remove malignant cells and other parasitic conditions, while toxicology is the study of harmful substances and how they affect the body, as well the study and discovery of remedies that will prevent such toxic effects. The first drug to be synthesized was morphine: in 1803, a Prussian pharmacist named Friedrich Serturner isolated morphine from opium.

There are many types of drugs to choose from when deciding what is needed for treatment; here is just a sampling of some of the main drug classes: analgesics, anesthetics, antibiotics, anticancer, anticoagulants, anticonvulsants, antidepressants, antidiabetics, antifungals, antihistamines, antivirals, cardiovascular, endocrine, gastrointestinal, sedatives, stimulants and tranquilizers. Picking the proper drug is crucial for successfully dealing with a specific health issue but an equally important consideration is deciding upon the correct potency. Drug potency, or the strength of the drug, is based upon the belief that there exists a specific dosage that will create the optimal therapeutic effect. This healing effect that a drug can produce is called drug efficacy.

To make certain that drugs are regulated and processed correctly, rules have been developed, and administrative oversight agencies have been established, dating back to the early twentieth century. In 1906, the Pure Food and Drug Act was passed and signed into law with the support of President Theodore Roosevelt. This Act went into effect on January 1, 1907, and required drug and food manufacturers in the United States to label their products correctly, with warnings if necessary, and to process them carefully prior to distribution, ensuring that no harmful substances had been added. In 1914, the Harrison Narcotics Tax Act passed and became a federal law. This law regulated and taxed the production, importation and distribution of opiates and cocaine. Also in 1914, the Federal Trade Commission Act gave the Federal Trade Commission the ability to declare "unfair methods of competition" to be unlawful. By 1938, to improve the enforcement of the Federal Trade Commission Act, the Wheeler-Lea Act passed and gave the Federal Trade Commission the ability to regulate drug, food and cosmetic advertising, in order to prevent misleading or false advertising. By 1970, the Controlled Substances Act was passed and signed by President Richard Nixon. This act provided that the Food and Drug Administration, or FDA, as well as the Drug Enforcement Administration, or DEA, regulate the manufacturing and distribution of drugs which can be harmful or damaging to the general public if not correctly prescribed. The drugs have five schedules for classification. Schedule I drugs have no known medical use in the U.S. and have a high potential for abuse. Examples are heroin and LSD. Schedule II drugs are accepted for medical use in the U.S. but are highly addictive and have a high potential for abuse. Examples are morphine, Ritalin, Concerta and cocaine. Schedule III drugs are also accepted for medical use in the U.S., may be moderately addictive and have less abusive potential than the Schedule I or II drugs. Examples are barbiturates such as Butisol and muscle-building steroids. Schedule IV drugs are fine for medical use, have a limited psychological or physical dependency and a low potential for abuse. Examples are Xanax and Valium. Schedule V drugs are accepted for medical use, the least likely to cause any type of addiction and have a low potential for abuse. Examples are antidiarrheals or over-the-counter medicines that contain codeine.

Having explored the history of drugs in the West, along with related considerations of potency, efficacy, safety and regulation, let's now look at how Chinese and Ayurvedic herbal medicines evolved and how they are utilized today.

Chinese and Ayurvedic herbal medicine consist of natural substances derived from a plant, mineral, shell or animal. The herbal ingredients are mixed together in very specific ratios to make a formula. The formula restores health by removing problematic symptoms and ailments while remaining balanced enough to minimize most side effects.

Chinese herbal medicine (as previously mentioned in Chapter

One) has a few historical highlights. More than 2000 years BCE, Shen Nong or the Divine Farmer, wrote *Pen T'sao* or *The Herbal*. This book is considered the first herbal medicinal text. Around 600 CE, Zhen Quan was not only busy revising medical texts for acupuncture and moxibustion, but also wrote *Yao Xing Ben Cao* or the *Materia Medica of Medicinal Properties*. Herbal medicinal knowledge especially expanded when Li Shizhen in 1578 wrote an encyclopedia of medicinal ingredients called the *Bencao Gangmu* or *Outlines of Roots and Herbs Studies*. Zhao Xuemin added to that extensive compilation, by writing about 921 more medicinal substances in *Bencao Gangmu Shiyi* or *Supplement to Compendium of Materia Medica*, first published in 1765. Currently, there is a very learned group of Chinese herbal scholars who have continued this tradition by translating these and other ancient herbal medical texts into as many languages as possible.

Chinese herbal medicine can be described according to its tastes and properties. The five main tastes are yin, and range from bitter or *ku*, sour or *suan*, sweet or *gan*, pungent or *xin* and salty or *xian*. Astringent or *se* herbs, and bland or *dan* herbs, also sometimes describe the taste of an herb. The function of bitter herbs is to detoxify, dry dampness, disperse stagnant qi and drain qi blockages. Sour herbs absorb, consolidate and astringe toxins that need to leave the body. (Astringent herbs are very similar to sour herbs so they are included in the sour category.) Sweet herbs tonify qi and can harmonize and balance formulas. (Bland herbs which are calming, soothing and diuretic in nature, are included in the sweet category.) Pungent herbs disperse qi and promote circulation while salty herbs soften and dissolve hardenings and can act as a purgative. The tastes also travel through the meridians and affect certain organs. Bitter herbs enter the heart, sour herbs the liver, sweet herbs the spleen, pungent herbs the lungs and salty herbs the kidney.

The properties, or temperatures, of herbs are yang, and range from hot or *re*, cold or *han,* warm or *wen,* cool or *liang,* neutral

or *ping,* slightly warm or *wei wan* and slightly cold or *wei han.*
Aromatic or *xiang* herbs belong with the temperature of herbs
rather than the taste description, and have the ability to clear
turbidity and awaken the spleen functions or the spirit. Both
herbal temperatures and tastes guide themselves and move along
the meridians to treat symptoms from imbalanced organs and
systems (both physiological and energetic). There are many
herbal categories, but here a few categories that created the
foundation for today's vast variety of herbs: promote sweating,
induce vomiting, purge, harmonize, warm, clear or cool, tonify
and reduce. When an herbal formula is created, it is with
the primary focus of their combined curative properties, but
consideration is also given to herbs that will prevent side effects.
This is what is meant by a formula that is "balanced."

Currently, Chinese herbs are being researched and studied
according to their pharmacodynamic and pharmacokinetic
interactions. Researchers are finding the active ingredient in
the herb, understanding how the herb is absorbed, metabolized
and eliminated, and how the herb affects tissues and organs in
the body. This crossover of study will benefit both herbal and
pharmacological medicines; perhaps one day soon, Western
drugs will be discussed according to their tastes, properties and
meridian connections.

Depending upon how an herb or formula is labelled and used,
they are classified as either a dietary supplement or drug. We
have already reviewed drug regulation specifications, so let's take
a brief look at dietary supplement regulation. In 1994, Congress
passed the Dietary Supplement Health and Education Act, or
DSHEA. This act defined a dietary supplement, required specific
product labelling, created a regulatory outline, and authorized the
FDA to regulate dietary supplements according to "GMP," or Good
Manufacturing Practices. Dietary supplements fall under the
general category of food. If an herb or formula is properly labelled
and does not make any drug claim, then it is a dietary supplement.
If an herb or formula is used for diagnosis, treatment, prevention

or cure of a disease, it falls under the category of a drug. Furthermore, in 2003, the FDA proposed rules for the CGMP, or Current Good Manufacturing Practices; these specified that regardless of where the product is in the distribution pipeline – manufacture, packing, storage, or actual sale – it needs to contain precisely what the manufacturer says it contains. The product also needs to be hygienic, free of contaminants or adulterations and must be accurately labelled. The above mentioned regulations are deemed necessary to ensure the highest quality of the herbs (Chinese, Ayurvedic or other) and formulas.

Whether during the time the Silk Road was travelled or when the Golden Age of India thrived, Chinese and Ayurvedic herbal medicinal information has been exchanged. What now follows are a few highlights from the ancient Ayurvedic herbal tradition (some of which was previously mentioned in Chapter One). The *Rig Veda,* the oldest written book, contains information about herbs and their curative powers. The *Yajur Veda* mentions how herbs are sacred and healing. Around 1300 CE, the *Sharangdhara Samhita,* written by Acharya Sharangdhara, contained important information about herbal and pharmacological formulas. Approximately 1500 CE, the *Bhava Prakasha,* authored by Bhava Mishra, described plant and mineral characteristics. Adding to the these contributions, Hendrik van Rheede, a Dutch colonial governor and naturalist, and his colleagues, in the period from 1686 to 1703, compiled *Hortus Malabaricus,* a twelve volume set that described around eight hundred Indian plants and their medicinal properties. Currently, Ayurvedic herbal medicine continues to expand its knowledge-base, and to share its findings globally.

Like Chinese herbal medicine, Ayurvedic herbal medicine uses taste and temperature to describe herbs. Ayurvedic herbal medicine additionally uses substance qualities for description. The six tastes for Ayurvedic herbs are sweet or *madhura,* sour or *amla,* salty or *lavana,* pungent or *katu,* bitter or *tikta*, and astringent or *kashaya*. These tastes have temperatures, substance qualities and herbal functions. Sweet herbs are cool, heavy, and oily, and one function is to nourish the body and mind. Sour herbs are hot, heavy, and oily, and a function example is to improve appetite and digestion. Salty herbs are hot, heavy, and oily, and one function is to cleanse the body. Pungent herbs are hot, light, dry and a function example is to improve the appetite. Bitter herbs are cool, light, dry and some functions are to control skin diseases and fevers. Astringent herbs are cool, light, dry and one function is to reduce glandular substances. Metals and minerals even have taste properties. For example, gold is sweet, silver is sour, copper is pungent and iron is astringent. Ayurvedic herbal remedies try to balance the doshas and this is the key to any formulation; this particular tradition, as part of its treatment, also relies on nutrition in achieving this same balance. Food, like herbs and pharmaceuticals, has been known since ancient times to have curative properties; this is one of the reasons why the next chapter will explore the various approaches to healthy nutrition from Western, Chinese and Ayurvedic perspectives. Using medication properly, whether herbal or pharmacological, is of the utmost importance. Be your own best advocate and read about the herbs and prescriptions you are using. Become educated by purchasing a *Physician's Desk Reference,* an herbal encyclopedia, or use the internet to acquire information about what you are ingesting. Know why you are taking particular powders, teas or pills. Also, be aware of side effects or possible contraindications. Pay attention to how your body feels after you have ingested either herbs or drugs. The following diary is intended as a template for journaling all of these important aspects of personal herbal and drug use. Visit **vitalityfusion.com** to print a copy of this diary and keep a record of your prescriptions and herbs.

Herbal and Pharmaceutical Diary

Herb or drug name, function, dosage, side effects, how you feel on the medicine

Aspirin decreases my headache pain. I take 1 or 2 tablets of 325 mg. Sometimes my stomach is irritated but mostly I feel clear and awake after the aspirin starts working.

Chapter Four:
Western, Chinese and Ayurvedic Nutrition

"Eat Good Food." - DR . E.F. KORMAN

Food is our fuel. To stay healthy, we must eat quality food. It sounds simple, but actually figuring out what to put in our mouths can be confusing and complex. Eating on the run is the norm, using caffeine to get through the day is a given, and dessert is an expected part of our everyday meal. To offset this intake, commercials advertise a new, yummy fat-free or sugar-free item, weight loss programs tout the latest miracle cure, and being twiggy-thin is the consensus goal of health and beauty.

Chinese and Ayurvedic nutrition therapies describe the function and nutritive aspects of food in a very different way than the Western model. The Western world analyzes food according to its biochemical structure. The ancient nutrition therapies look at the taste of food as well as what effect it will have on the energy of the body; this energetic approach is consistent with the non-Western herbal medicine philosophies surveyed in Chapter Three.

At the end of this chapter, there will be another personal

exercise intended to help explore the relevance of these different traditions in your own life, in your own quest for balance and good health. A food diary will help you to record and analyze your own eating habits. Becoming aware of these habits is the first step to understanding not just the best things to eat, but the best way to ingest them. But let's first start with a review of the Western school of nutritional theory and practice.

In order for the body to receive its nutrients, the process of digestion and metabolism must first occur. Digestion is how food moves through the body, and this process begins in the mouth. As food is ingested, saliva containing important enzymes is released on each side of the mouth. These enzymes are substances that quicken the chemical reactions that break down the ingested food. From the mouth, food travels down the esophagus with help from involuntary movement, called peristalsis. From the esophagus, food then moves to the stomach.

Here, hydrochloric acid, along with enzymes such as pepsin and digestive hormones such as gastrin, prepare the food mechanically and chemically to travel in minute amounts to the small intestine. The small intestine has three parts. The first part, the duodenum, receives food from the stomach, bile from the liver and gallbladder, and pancreatic juice from the pancreas. The second part, the jejunum, connects with the third part, the ileum, which attaches to the beginning of the large intestine. Tiny blood vessels in microscopic protuberances called villi pass digested nutrients into the bloodstream and lymph vessels.

The large intestine receives the fluid waste products of digestion that did not pass into the bloodstream. These products are stored until the large intestine can release them from the body. Water in the wastes is absorbed through the walls of the large intestine while solid stools are formed. The four parts to the large intestine are the cecum, colon (ascending, transverse and descending), sigmoid colon and rectum.

The duodenum previously mentioned connects with the liver. The liver produces fluid called bile. Bile contains cholesterol, bile acids and several bile pigments, in particular, bilirubin. Bile breaks apart large fat globules so the pancreas can digest them. Without this process, most fat would remain undigested. Bile travels to the gallbladder to regulate its usage. The liver also regulates blood sugar, manufactures blood proteins, destroys old red blood cells and detoxifies the blood.

The pancreas also connects with the duodenum. The pancreas produces pancreatic juices filled with the enzyme amylase, for digesting starch, and lipase, for digesting fats. The pancreas also produces insulin. Insulin releases sugar from the blood to be used for energy by the body.

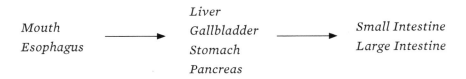

Mouth
Esophagus

Liver
Gallbladder
Stomach
Pancreas

Small Intestine
Large Intestine

Digestion describes how food travels through the body; metabolism is the cellular process that converts this food into energy. The metabolic process is itself a combination of anabolism and catabolism. Anabolism builds up complex materials from simple materials, while catabolism breaks down complex materials to form simpler substances and release energy. Metabolism works with macronutrients such as proteins, fats, carbohydrates, micronutrients such as vitamins and minerals and one of the most important bodily nutrients, water. After the metabolic process has finished, the unwanted products are excreted as urine, feces, sweat and exhaled carbon dioxide. Let's now take a closer look at those macronutrients – proteins, fats and carbohydrates.

Protein is a macronutrient that is found in every cell, tissue and organ of our body, and is essential for growth and development.

When protein is metabolized, it is broken down into building blocks called amino acids. Amino acids are either essential or non-essential. Essential amino acids, such as lysine and tryptophan, cannot be made by our body so they must come from our diet. Meats, poultry, dairy, nuts and beans are good sources. Non-essential amino acids, such as arginine and taurine, can be put together by our body. Protein examples are described below.

Protein Sources

Milk, dairy products and eggs

Meat, poultry, fish

Nuts and seeds

Dry beans and peas

Rice with beans

Another macronutrient is fat. Fat insulates and cushions the body, creates the most concentrated form of energy, carries fat soluble vitamins, regulates the hunger mechanism and holds onto food flavor. Fats are composed of building blocks called fatty acids. The three main types of fatty acids are saturated, polyunsaturated and monounsaturated. Saturated fats are found in animal and dairy products, and are what the liver uses to manufacture a type of fatty substance called cholesterol. Polyunsaturated fats are primarily found in oils, such as corn and safflower oil. Monounsaturated fats are found in vegetables and nut oils, like olive and canola oil. Examples of fat products are listed below.

Fat Sources

Oils, salad dressings

Butter, margarine

Bacon, meat or poultry with fat attached

Egg yolks

To determine the fat content of a food item, look at the total number of fat grams per serving of the product and multiply by 9. Next, divide that amount by the total number of calories per serving, to find out the fat percentage (grams x 9 / calories = fat percentage). For example, if the food has 5 grams of fat per serving, then multiply 5 times 9 to get an answer or 45. Next, if the calories per serving is 150, divide 150 by 45, for an answer of .3 or 30 percent fat.

Another way to notice how much fat is in a product is to check product labels. A few of the common fat descriptions are given below.

Fat Free   *less than .5 grams of fat per serving*

Low Fat   *3 grams or less of fat per serving*

Lean   *less than 10 grams of fat*

Light/"Lite"   *50 percent less fat or 1/3 less calories than the regular product*

Cholesterol Free   *less than 2 milligrams of cholesterol per serving*

Carbohydrates are the other macronutrient that supplies energy for the body. There are two types of carbohydrates, simple and complex. The simple carbohydrates, or simple sugars, are typically fruit. The complex carbohydrates are considered fiber and starches, typically vegetables, grains and beans. Simple and complex carbohydrates (except for fiber) convert into blood glucose. Blood glucose is the fuel or energy for the brain, red blood cells and body's cells. A summary of common carbohydrate sources follows.

Carbohydrate Sources

Whole grain cereal, bread, pasta

Vegetables, potatoes

Fruit

No nutritional survey would be complete without a discussion of the role of fiber in our diet. Fiber is the name given to the indigestible portion of food from plants: it can either be soluble, and dissolve in water, or insoluble, and not dissolve in water. Fiber is important because it maintains normal elimination, maintains blood sugar levels, lowers blood cholesterol levels and fills you up, so you won't feel hungry too soon after your last meal. In the 1970's, Denis Burkitt, M.D., a British physician, observed during the course of his medical studies and experiences in Africa, that his native patients ate huge amounts of fiber as part of their traditional diet. By eating high-fiber foods, these native patients had low rates of numerous illnesses, such as constipation and colon cancer. Such was not the case with Europeans and natives who ate the European diet with processed foods. A few common fiber sources are included below.

Fiber Sources

Whole grains like bran

Fruits, especially seeded types

Vegetables

Legumes like beans and nuts

Now that we have discussed the macronutrients, let's turn our attention to the micronutrients, vitamins and minerals, which are also essential for health. The history of vitamins in the West begins with William Fletcher, an English doctor, who in 1905 was researching the cause of Beriberi. He discovered that eating unpolished rice prevented Beriberi while eating polished rice did not. He surmised that the husk of the rice must have contained special nutrients. Then, in 1912, Cashmir Funk, a Polish scientist, isolated compounds found in thiamine from rice husks. He named these special nutrients "vitamine" for "vita" meaning life and "amine" for the thiamine compounds. Vitamine was later shortened to vitamin because all the compounds were not amines. Vitamins are important for the specific body functions of growth, maintenance and reproduction and are classified as either water soluble or fat soluble. Let's look at common vitamins and some of their functions.

Vitamin A is fat soluble, acts as an antioxidant and enhances immunity, helps with the formation of bones and teeth, prevents night blindness and other eye conditions, is needed for skin repair, reduces acne, and slows the aging process. Some good sources of Vitamin A are green leafy and yellow vegetables, fish liver oils, whole milk and eggs.

Vitamin D is fat soluble, important for calcium and phosphorous metabolism, needed for growth, helps with development of the bones and teeth in children, and enhances immunity. Some good sources of Vitamin D are fish liver oils, milk, eggs, sweet potatoes and vegetable oils.

Vitamin E is fat soluble, acts an antioxidant, helpful in preventing cancer and cardiovascular disease, needed for tissue repair, reduces scarring with some wounds, relaxes leg cramps, and maintains healthy nerves and muscles. Good sources of Vitamin E are dark green leafy vegetables, nuts, seeds whole grains and vegetable oils.

Vitamin K is fat soluble and important for bone formation and repair, needed for prothrombin, which is essential for blood clotting, and helps convert glucose into glycogen for storage in the liver. Some sources of Vitamin K are spinach, collard greens, broccoli, oats, rye and safflower oil.

All of the B vitamins are water soluble and help to maintain healthy muscles, nerves, skin, eyes, hair and brain function.

Vitamin B-1 or Thiamine, is primarily important for carbohydrate metabolism. Good sources of thiamine are brown rice, fish, liver pork, poultry, asparagus and whole grains.

Vitamin B-2 or Riboflavin, is necessary for cell respiration and growth, red blood cell formation, helps with metabolism of carbohydrates, fats and proteins, aids in the prevention and treatment of cataracts and reduces dandruff. Riboflavin sources are whole grains, legumes, yogurt, cheese, meats, poultry and green vegetables.

Vitamin B-3 or Niacin, Niacinamide or Nicotinic Acid, helps the nervous system function, promotes healthy skin and proper circulation, lowers cholesterol and improves the memory. Sources are whole wheat, pork, fish, tomatoes, dandelion greens and dates.

Vitamin B-5 or Pantothenic Acid, is required by all cells in the body, helps to produce adrenal hormones and neurotransmitters, aids in vitamin processes and enhances the body's stamina. Food sources are fresh vegetables, legumes, nuts, beef, whole rye flour or whole wheat.

Vitamin B-6 or Pyridoxine, is important for many body functions such as helping normal brain function, aids in red blood cell formation, maintains a sodium and potassium balance, activates enzymes and improves immunity and cardiovascular health. Food sources are avocado, bananas, spinach and brown rice.

Vitamin B-12 or Cyanocobalamin, is needed to prevent anemia and help utilize iron and form red blood cells properly. Some primary food sources of vitamin B-12 are brewer's yeast, dairy products, eggs, liver and clams.

Vitamin C or Ascorbic Acid, is water soluble, and an antioxidant that promotes healthy gums and healing of wounds, protects against bruising, necessary for tissue growth and repair, helps to form collagen and supports adrenal gland function. Vitamin C sources are strawberries, citrus fruits, persimmons, green leafy vegetables, broccoli and brussel sprouts.

Vitamin P or Bioflavanoids, are water soluble, enhance the absorption of Vitamin C and need to be taken together. They are helpful with athletic injuries and relieve pain, bumps, and bruises. Bioflavanoids also have an antibacterial effect and promote circulation. A good source of these vitamins are cherries, apricots, lemons and oranges.

Folic Acid is water soluble, and needed for the formation of red blood cells and energy production, making white blood cells and strengthening immunity. Folic acid is important during pregnancy to regulate nerve cell formation of the baby. Sources of folic acid are green leafy vegetables, beef, brewer's yeast, milk and whole grain grains.

Coenzyme Q10 or Ubiquinone, is fat soluble, and a powerful antioxidant that enhances the immune system and slows the aging process. Food sources are salmon, beef and spinach.

Vitamins and minerals both help the body perform the activities of energy production, growth and healing. Let's now take a closer look at why minerals are beneficial. Minerals help to form blood and bone, regulate muscle tone, balance body fluids and maintain healthy nerve function. Minerals are grouped as either bulk or trace. Some of the common minerals are described below.

Calcium, a bulk mineral, is vital for the transmission of nerve impulses, growing strong bones and teeth, regulating the contraction and relaxation of muscles, including the heartbeat, and aiding in the clotting of blood. Good food sources are green leafy vegetables, salmon and dairy products.

Magnesium, a bulk mineral, is essential for all living cells. It is involved in enzyme activation for energy production, nerve impulse transmission and muscle relaxation. Food sources include dairy products, fish, meat, bananas, apples, brown rice, millet, nuts, green leafy vegetables and kelp.

Phosphorus, a bulk mineral, has many functions and is needed for converting food to energy, bone and tooth formation, cell growth and contraction of the heart muscle. Phosphorus is found in many foods, in particular, asparagus, dried fruit, eggs, dairy products and pumpkin seeds.

Potassium, a bulk mineral, aids in proper muscle contraction, keeps the nervous system healthy, prevents stroke, helps to provide a regular heart rhythm and stabilizes blood pressure. Good food sources are fruit, vegetables, legumes, fish, poultry, meat, dairy products and whole grains.

Sodium, a bulk mineral, is important for stomach, nerve and muscle function and for maintaining proper water balance and blood pH. Also, sodium and potassium need to be balanced for good health. Sodium is found in most foods.

Iron, a trace mineral, produces hemoglobin, myoglobin and oxygenates red blood cells. Iron helps with energy production and growth and maintaining a healthy immune system. Good food sources include green leafy vegetables, enriched bread, cereals and whole grains, eggs, fish and dates.

Zinc, a trace mineral, promotes a healthy immune system, heals wounds, reduces acne, supports the prostate gland function and reproductive organ growth, needed for protein synthesis and collagen formation. Some food sources are brewer's yeast, pecans, pumpkin seeds, lima beans, fish, eggs, kelp, mushrooms and whole grains.

Copper, a trace mineral, is essential in the formation of red blood cells, bone, healthy nerves and joints. Sources of food are barley, beans, almonds, raisins, oranges and green leafy vegetables.

Chromium, a trace mineral, helps the body use insulin efficiently and is needed for the synthesis of cholesterol, fats, and protein. Food sources that contain chromium are brown rice, brewer's yeast, cheese and meat.

We have now reviewed all of the macronutrients and micronutrients associated with metabolism. The last component, and arguably the most important, is water. Water makes up sixty-five percent of our body and is very essential to our existence. Water supports and cushions all cells, transports nutrients including water soluble vitamins, removes waste materials from the body and helps to maintain body temperature.

The American public has been aware for quite some time that eating enough good food to acquire sufficient amounts of each of these many nutritional components is a challenge. Consideration of the depletion of quality food sources is evident in a 1936 U.S. Senate Document, number 264 of the 74th Congress, Second Session, "Farm soils are depleted of minerals and crops, grains, vegetables, nuts grown on these farms are mineral deficient and the people who eat them get mineral deficiency diseases." More recently, Dr. Joel Wallach, an American medical doctor and veterinarian has commented, "the body needs 90 nutrients in your body everyday. The body needs 60 minerals, 16 vitamins, 12 essential amino acids and 3 essential fatty acids."

Stepping back from the detail of the Western nutritional survey and historical record for just a minute, and focusing more on matters of personal nutrition from this same Western perspective, finding the proper food to eat and deciding what additional vitamins and minerals your body might need is a challenge for all of us, regardless of our cultural heritage. We need to individually evaluate how our bodies are digesting, absorbing and metabolizing those nutrients we have discussed. Signs of healthy digestion include feeling alert and satisfied after eating, without bloating, gas, acid regurgitation, a stuffed feeling, fatigue, cramping or diarrhea. It is important to realize that these are all signs and symptoms of indigestion and are indications that our bodies are not truly absorbing much needed nutrition or fuel. How does one, in a Western nutritional environment, address any such digestive imbalances? We are bombarded with potential solutions. Dieting in the West is a big business: there are diets for balancing, detoxifying or losing weight; they range from combining food properly, eating monochromatic meals, ingesting a macrobiotic menu, feeding on a 40% carbohydrate with 30% fat and 30% protein plan, consuming a high carbohydrate and low-fat plan or eating a low carbohydrate with a ketosis- producing diet. Food programs can be designed according to a restricted calorie intake, blood type or hormonal body type. There are also many detoxification programs that treat yeast overgrowth, bacteria or parasites.

Now that we have looked at Western nutrition from the perspective of the human body, let's take a look at how nutrition has been affected by the body politic, specifically through the evolution of regulations and government guidelines. There are many government agencies that help to protect our food: the FDA, the EPA, the National Marine Fisheries Service within the U.S. Department of Commerce and the Bureau of Alcohol, Tobacco, Firearms and Explosives within the Department of Justice and last, but certainly not least, the USDA.

The Food and Drug Administration, or FDA, ensures the safety and quality of all food sold in interstate commerce except meat, poultry, and eggs. The FDA regulates food additives, sets legal limits for drug residues in milk, eggs, raw meat and poultry, regulates pesticide residues in food, tests food for contaminants and pesticide except for meat and poultry and regulates labelling of food except for meat, poultry and eggs.

The Environmental Protection Agency, or EPA, is responsible for approving the use and application levels of pesticides and setting tolerance levels for pesticide residues in foods. These levels are enforced by the FDA. The EPA sets national drinking-water standards for public drinking water supplies.

The National Oceanic and Atmospheric Administration, or NOAA, within the U.S. Department of Commerce, uses the National Marine Fisheries Service for a fee, to voluntarily inspect a portion of the seafood consumed in the United States.

The Bureau of Alcohol, Tobacco, Firearms and Explosives, or ATF, within the Department of Justice, oversees the labelling of alcoholic beverages and regulates the use of FDA-approved additives in alcoholic beverages.

The final entry in this list of acronym-agencies, and, from the perspective of food regulation, certainly one of the most important, is the previously mentioned United States Department of Agriculture or USDA. The USDA is responsible for the safety of meat, poultry, and eggs sold through interstate commerce. The USDA's Food Safety and Inspection Service, or FSIS, is responsible for inspecting meat and poultry products and regulates food and color additives in meat and poultry; and its Agriculture Marketing Service, or AMS, inspects eggs and egg products, and sets the national standards for organic food. The United States Department of Agriculture has also been making food recommendations for the United States since 1916. The USDA's first food guide, "Food for Young Children" by nutritionist Caroline Hunt, put food into five classifications. The groupings were cereals, vegetables and fruit, milk and meat, fats and fatty foods and sugars and sugary foods. Since that time, the U.S. government routinely tries to advise the American public what an overall healthy diet entails with "The Dietary Guidelines for Americans." These guidelines are presented by the Department of Health and Human Services, or HHS, and the USDA. They are updated every five years. In 1992, the USDA provided these food recommendations in the form of a pyramid with four tiers. The

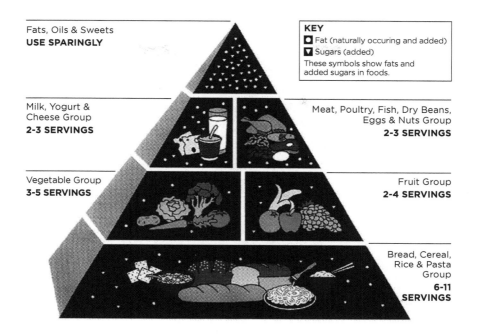

Fats, Oils & Sweets
USE SPARINGLY

KEY
◻ Fat (naturally occuring and added)
▼ Sugars (added)
These symbols show fats and
added sugars in foods.

Milk, Yogurt &
Cheese Group
2-3 SERVINGS

Meat, Poultry, Fish, Dry Beans,
Eggs & Nuts Group
2-3 SERVINGS

Vegetable Group
3-5 SERVINGS

Fruit Group
2-4 SERVINGS

Bread, Cereal,
Rice & Pasta
Group
**6-11
SERVINGS**

bottom tier suggested a group of bread, cereal, rice and pasta with
6-11 servings, the next to the bottom tier suggested vegetables
with 3-5 servings and a fruit group of 2-4 servings, the next to the
top tier put milk, yogurt and cheeses with 2-3 servings and meat,
fish, poultry, dry beans, eggs and nuts at 2-3 servings and the top
tier recommended that fats, oils and sweets are sparingly used.

The USDA's most recent guidelines, released January 31, 2011,
state three main dietary goals. First, balance calories with physical
activity. Second, consume more of certain foods and nutrients
such as fruits, vegetables, whole grains, fat-free and low-fat dairy
products, and seafood. Lastly, consume fewer foods with sodium
(salt), saturated fats, transfats, cholesterol, added sugars, and
refined grains. (Doesn't this sound a lot like the USDA's first food
guide, "Food for Young Children" in 1916? If there seems to be
one recurring theme in this chapter, it is Dr. Korman's dictum to
"eat good food.") As of June, 2011, the USDA's 1992 food pyramid
has been replaced with a USDA food plate. The plate has four
sections: fruits, vegetables, grains and proteins, with a small side
of dairy. This simple breakdown of what our meal plates ought

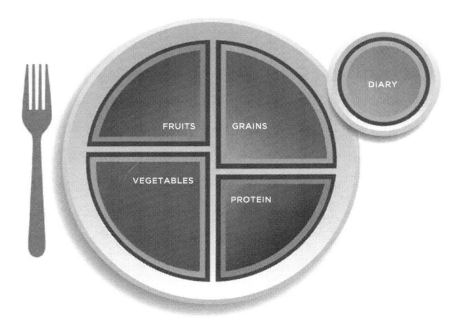

choosemyplate.gov

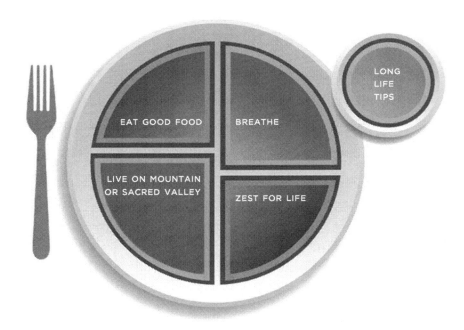

Longevity Plate

to look like at breakfast, lunch or dinner, will be helpful when preparing meals in our homes. The plate is intended to make it easier to remember how to prepare healthy meals and encourage more nutritious eating habits.

All of these U.S. agencies are trying to help and provide optimum food and water so people can live a long time. While these services continue to improve the quality and safety of our nutrition, let's mention some other cultures where people live a very long time, ranging approximately from 120 to 140 years. One of them exists in the mountainous area of Tibet, China, where the culture is characterized by simple living and great longevity. A famous doctor, Li Chung-Yun, lived approximately 200 to 250 years from around 1677 to 1933. The Imperial government even gave him a certificate award after living 150 years. Other long-living groups of people are the Georgians and Armenians, from the Caucasus Mountains between Europe and Asia. These people have a unique zest for life. Yet another select group, the Vilcabamba people from Ecuador, reside in a sacred valley along the Andes Mountains, breathing some of the purest air on the planet. Below the USDA food plate is a longevity plate based on some of the attributes of these cultures, suggesting the best way to live a happy and long life.

There are elements in this longevity plate that have not appeared in any USDA publication; yet, these elements touch on aspects of nutrition that have been common in Chinese and Ayurvedic guidelines for centuries. Let's explore some of these differences as we start with a survey of Chinese medicine's approach to nutrition.

Chinese medicine states that the only way that we can fuel our bodies is from the air we breathe and the food we eat. That's it. Most of us don't have the type of control over the air we breathe, that we do with the daily food choices we make. If your car doesn't have the proper fuel, it will stop working or drive sluggishly. It is no different for our bodies. Nature is available for our nutrition, and Chinese medicine wants us to respect and use this gift, while at the same time optimizing our health.

Chinese medicine describes food according to its specific tastes, the effect the taste has when travelling through the meridian or element, and temperature of the food. The five tastes are sour, bitter, sweet, pungent and salty. Sour travels to the liver and gallbladder meridians or wood element, bitter goes to the heart and small intestine energy pathways or fire element, sweet travels to the spleen and stomach meridians or earth element, pungent goes to the lung and large intestine energy pathways or metal element and salty goes to the kidney and urinary bladder meridians or water element.

Taste	Meridian	Element	Function	Food
SOUR	LIVER, GALL BLADDER	WOOD	ASTRINGING, ABSORBING	BITTER MELONS, KALE
BITTER	HEART, SMALL INTESTINE	FIRE	DRYING, DESCENDING	LEMONS, VINEGAR
SWEET	SPLEEN, STOMACH	EARTH	NOURISHING, EXPANDING	YAMS, CARROTS
PUNGENT	LUNG, LARGE INTESTINE	METAL	STIMULATING, DISPERSING	GINGER, ONIONS
SALTY	KIDNEY, URINARY BLADDER	WATER	SOFTENING, CONCENTRATING	SEAWEED, CLAMS

Using the Five Element theory to decide food choices, according to Chinese medicine, has its benefits. One picks the appropriate food to nourish that element, or the food to calm and sedate the hyperactive element. Following are some meat, fruit, vegetables, grains and nut items described according to their element.

	Wood	Fire	Earth	Metal	Water
Meat	CHICKEN	LAMB	BEEF	DUCK	PORK
Fruit	PLUM	WATERMELON	DATES	PEAR	RASPBERRY
Veggie	LEEKS	LOTUS ROOT	CUCUMBER	ASPARAGUS	SWEET POTATO
Grain	WHEAT	CORN	WHITE RICE	BUCKWHEAT	MILLET
Nut	SESAME SEEDS	LOTUS SEED	CHESTNUT	ALMONDS	WALNUTS

The five food temperatures are hot, warm, neutral, cool and cold. Here is a list of the temperatures with some corresponding foods and spices.

Hot	*Warm*	*Neutral*	*Cool*	*Cold*
LAMB	CHERRY	CELERY	BUCKWHEAT	SALT
DRIED GINGER	SQUASH	RYE	SESAME OIL	CRAB
PEPPER	SWEET RICE	ALMONDS	EGG WHITE	GRAPEFRUIT
CINNAMON BARK	WALNUT	BEEF	APPLE	ROMAINE LETTUCE
COTTONSEED	CHICKEN	APRICOT	SPINACH	CLAMS

It is an interesting concept to first determine your body temperature, or what organs, meridians or elements within your body may not be in balance, as a precursor to deciding your meal choices. If your body is cold, eat warm food; if your lung is weak, you may want to eat something pungent such as onions; if your liver is overstressed, you may want to avoid ingesting foods that travel to the liver like chicken. If you are craving something sweet, you might eat a date or carrot to nourish your body. Depending upon the amount of imbalance in your system, you may need to eat foods that will detoxify the excesses and, then afterwards, eat foods that will strengthen and harmonize the depleted organs or energies.

Food choices are also eaten according to the seasons. In the spring, it is a good time to detoxify and "spring clean" your body by giving your liver a rest. In the summer, it is a good time to stay cool and not overwork your heart with all the outdoor heat and summer fun, so watermelon and corn-on-the-cob provide some balance. Other choices are persimmons, crab apples, egg yolks and adzuki or mung beans. During autumn, when it is the best time to harvest fabulous food and also fortify your lungs, eating pumpkin, sweet potatoes, asparagus, mandarin oranges, pears, duck, peanuts and almonds is recommended. In the winter, whether your body is faced with cold outside temperatures or an extreme amount of holiday activities, it is important to keep your kidney energy strong and vital. You might want to roast chestnuts on an open fire, enjoy plum pudding or drink hot chocolate with some cinnamon spice added. These would be good choices to support your kidney, along with eating lamb, pork, shrimp, string beans and millet. Also during the winter, because heavy and rich food have been consumed, either because of the cold weather or the many celebrations during that time of year, the body can be cleansed with a diet of celery, leeks, raspberries, pine nuts, sesame seeds and whole wheat.

A pot of boiling water with rice inside, and a flame below the pot continuing to cook the rice, is an important image to remember when picturing healthy digestion in Chinese medicine. The water and fire work together to cook the rice. The water is the kidney energy, the fire is the heart energy, and the rice is the spleen energy. Nicely cooked rice means the spleen is healthy and digestion is functioning well. Digestion is focused on the spleen organ and meridian because it must transform and transport food nutrients to be distributed as qi and blood. The spleen governs all digestive activities from the mouth to the large intestine, even the liver, gallbladder and pancreas. The spleen is the control center, and signals the nutritious qi and pure food essence to mix with the air from the lungs and then head to the appropriate meridians and organs for digestion. The turbid particles are also earmarked and transported to the stomach, small intestine, kidney, urinary bladder and large intestine to be separated and eliminated. This digestive process can be impeded if the foods consumed are unhealthy, if there is too much stress when eating, or if you wait too long before eating or overeat. When you feel uncomfortable, it is a good time to pause and consider the taste, energetic function, temperature and seasonal timing of the food. Like a car that is beginning to consistently drift to one side of the road, this is a signal that your body needs to be rebalanced by finding a better alignment of what it needs and the taste and energetic function, temperature and season of the food you are consuming.

In this respect, Chinese nutritional advice is very similar to its Ayurvedic "cousin" - Ayurvedic nutrition would offer some of the same suggestions, especially in regard to the taste and energetic qualities of food and their effect on the doshas (explained in greater detail below). Let's take a look at some of the other similarities and differences associated with Ayurvedic nutritional guidance.

There are six tastes to describe food in Ayurvedic nutrition: sweet, salty, sour, pungent, astringent and bitter. Sweet is mostly a combination of the earth and water elements and the sweet taste nourishes body tissues and enhances the mind. The sweet qualities are cooling, heavy and oily. Salty is primarily a combination of the water and fire elements and the salty taste helps to eliminates wastes and cleanse the body and also provides a proper mineral balance in the body. The salty qualities are heavy, heating and oily. The sour taste is mostly a combination of the earth and fire elements and it improves the appetite, digestion and lessens spasms and tremors. The sour qualities are heating, heavy and oily. The pungent taste is primarily a combination of the fire and air elements and improves the appetite, removes secretions from the body and reduces fat. The pungent qualities are heating, light and dry. The astringent taste is mainly a combination of the air and earth elements and heals and purifies the body. The astringent qualities are cooling, light and dry. The bitter taste is primarily a combination of the air and ether elements; it detoxifies the body, controls skin diseases and fevers, strengthens the immune system and returns all the tastes to a normal balance. The bitter qualities are cooling, light and dry.

These tastes will balance the biological humors, known as doshas, if eaten correctly. Let's look at what tastes and foods work for the vata, pitta and kapha body types.

Recommended tastes for a vata are sweet, sour and salty while bitter, astringent and pungent tastes are not encouraged. Grains, dairy and nuts are beneficial for a vata.

Recommended tastes for a pitta body type are bitter, astringent and sweet and sour, salty and pungent tastes are not advised. Raw vegetables, in particular large salads, are beneficial for a pitta.

Suggested tastes for a kapha body type are pungent, bitter and astringent flavors while sweet, sour and salty flavors are advised to be avoided. Cooked vegetables, buckwheat and millet grains and pungent foods are beneficial for a kapha.

Lists for suggested foods for the vata, pitta and kapha body types follow.

Vata Food List

Grains such as oats and rice

Cooked vegetables such as carrots and asparagus

Avoid nightshade vegetables

Most fruits except dried fruits

Animal protein, but reduce the amount of red meat

Lentils, chickpeas or mung beans

Almonds or pumpkin seeds

Sesame, almond, coconut and mustard oil

All dairy

Occasional sweeteners but no white sugar

Spices are good

Pitta Food List

Barley, rice, oats, wheat

Leafy green vegetables, broccoli, asparagus, potatoes

Avoid tomatoes, radishes, garlic

Sweet fruit like grapes, mangos, cherries, not sour fruit

Chicken, turkey, venision

Chickpeas, mung beans, tofu

Coconut, sunflower and pumpkin seeds

Milk and ghee but avoid sour cream and yogurt

Sweeteners except molasses and avoid mustard and salt

Kapha Food List

Buckwheat, millet, barley, rice, corn

All vegetables except tomatoes, potatoes and water chestnuts

Dried prunes, apples, pears or apricots

Eggs, seafood, chicken

Mung beans, black and pinto beans, red lentils

Avoid nuts except pumpkin and sunflower seeds on occasion

Avoid oils except safflower and almond on occasion

Avoid dairy except small amounts of ghee and goat milk

No sweeteners except raw honey and all spices except salt

Eat according to the dosha suggestions, but also check and see if there are any excesses or deficiencies in the body. If needed, purifying and cleansing, calming, rejuvenating and tonifying therapies are used to balance the doshas.

As is the case with Chinese nutrition, dietary requirements can also change according to the seasons. For example, during the spring, lighter grains, spring vegetables and sprouts, juices and cleansing herbs are recommended. In the summer, the food suggestions are millet, quinoa, rice and corn along with fresh fruits and vegetables. In the fall, the optimum diet would include harvest grains, pumpkins, legumes, squash, seeds and nuts. And finally, during the winter, heavier grains, green leafy vegetables, legumes, roots, seeds and nuts are recommended.

In the Ayurvedic explanation of digestion, taste is what your body first registers before digestive process actually begins. This taste, or *rasa,* occurs in the mouth and mixes with saliva and the alkaline secretions of the stomach. This process is considered the kapha stage. Next energy, or *virya,* is produced to digest food. Food nutrients are metabolized, harmful substances are detoxified and prana is extracted from the food. This process involves the small intestine and liver, and is considered the pitta stage. After digestion, the post-digestive effect, or *vipaka,* absorbs important nutrients while the colon eliminates waste. This is considered the vata stage.

No matter what you decide for your next meal, it is a general consensus within both the ancient and modern nutritional traditions that you eat in an inviting and calm environment, that you chew your food completely and enjoy the tastes of your meal, that you eat the freshest food possible and, finally, that you not try to stuff yourself. Pay attention before, during and after digesting a meal, to determine just how you feel physiologically, mentally, emotionally and spiritually. Are you energized, clear headed, centered and grateful for the delicious meal you just ingested? If the answer is yes, then you have obtained the goal of a healthy meal plate. If the answer is no, keep a record of your food intake. Visit **vitalityfusion.com** and print the food diary which follows to chart your meals, feelings and environment when eating. The diary will help you become more aware of what nutritional changes may be needed to help you feel your best. The next chapter will explore Western, Chinese and Ayurvedic exercise and will be another way to help you become aware of your physical, mental, emotional and spiritual well-being. Ways to increase your energy and improve your overall physical health will be discussed.

Food Diary

Date	Time	My Experience Eating (snacks, lunch...)	How I feel after the meal
	7am	Do I chew slowly?	Energized?
		Do I inhale food?	Bloated?
		Do I enjoy eating?	Bad Breath?
		Do I feel rushed when eating?	Satisfied?
		Is where I eat peaceful?	Sleepy?
		Is where I eat noisy?	Still craving?
		Do I eat a variety of food?	Sinuses congest?

7am –breakfast with coffee and cereal, banana and milk. I eat quickly and feel energized.

_____
_____
_____
_____
_____
_____
_____
_____
_____
_____
_____
_____
_____
_____
_____
_____
_____
_____
_____
_____
_____
_____
_____
_____

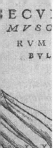

Chapter Five:
Western, Chinese and
Ayurvedic Exercise

"The sovereign invigorator of the body is exercise,
and of all the exercises walking is the best."
-THOMAS JEFFERSON

This chapter looks at the various ways that Western, Chinese and Ayurvedic cultures view exercise, describes their corresponding body types, and ends with an introduction of my own exercise philosophy with a program that synthesizes different aspects of each of these traditions. These exercises are simple and unique and have been successfully used for the last two decades in my wellness practice.

Since prehistoric days, man has needed to be fit in order to survive and prosper in his environment. Hunting, gathering and farming were the original exercise programs. As civilizations evolved, physical fitness routines and philosophy developed with them. Western exercise regimens date back to the ancient Greeks, including Hippocrates, who idolized physical perfection and realized that a strong, healthy body was necessary for a sound mind. The Romans exercised to prepare for the military while during the Middle Ages, people exercised to survive. During the Renaissance, people realized, like the Greeks, that a high fitness level enhanced intellectual learning. Fitness training and its value continued to grow and strengthen as America began to grow in the 1700's, so much so that physical activity became a staple along with other survival basics. Thomas Jefferson was a firm believer in fitness training. "Not less than two hours a day should be devoted to exercise, and the weather shall be little regarded. If the body is feeble, the mind will not be strong."

In America, after the Great Depression, Jack LaLanne, considered the "Godfather of Fitness," opened up the nation's first modern health studio in 1936. By the early 1950's, his exercise regimes were some of the first programs to be televised to millions of Americans. He emphasized that exercise builds confidence, allows one to feel "vim and vigor," improves the function of all the internal organs, enhances mental abilities, speeds up circulation, and improves coordination and balance, especially when combined with weight training. His memorable philosophy for longevity was "Exercise is king, nutrition is queen, put them together and you have a kingdom." By 1968, Dr. Kenneth Cooper, considered "the Father of the Modern Fitness Movement" influenced many people to exercise for preventative reasons. He called his program Aerobics. This program emphasized pumping oxygen while moving. Dr. Cooper found data to support the benefits of his new aerobic exercise program: the data showed that aerobic exercise prevented chronic diseases and helped to maintain a high level of fitness throughout life.

On July 11, 1996, the Surgeon General released a report on physical activity and health. This report was prepared by the Centers for Disease Control, or CDC, and other academic experts. The Surgeon General emphasized two findings. One finding stated that health benefits occur at a "moderate" level of activity- a level sufficient to expend about 150 calories of energy per day, or 1000 calories per week (e.g., walking briskly for 30 minutes each day). The second finding stated that while physical activity does not need to be vigorous to provide health benefits, the amount of health benefit is directly related to the amount of regular physical activity. These moderate exercise recommendations seem flexible and reasonable even for the busiest person or for someone who doesn't enjoy exercise. In 2010, the Gallup poll reported that 51.1% of Americans exercised for at least 30 minutes three or more days a week. Also in 2010, the Centers for Disease Control and Prevention's guidelines suggested adults get at least 150 minutes of "moderate-intensity aerobic activity" per week or 75 minutes of "vigorous-intensity aerobic activity."

Exercise is more important and popular than ever and exercise options are quite varied today. A walk in the park, hiking in the mountains, running, kayaking, swimming, bicycling, aerobic classes, strength and weight training classes, boot camps for shaping up, dance and pilates classes, and yoga and martial art classes are just a few examples of what people currently do for activity. According to the National Sporting Goods Association, or NSGA, the top five sports that Americans participated in during 2010 were yoga, aerobic exercising, tennis, hiking and running/jogging.

To help determine which exercise you may prefer, it is useful to first understand your body type. There are three Western body types, or somatotypes. According to Dr. William Herbert Sheldon, an American psychologist, body types can be described as ectomorph, mesomorph or endomorph.

Illustrations for each of these body types follow.

Ectomorph

The ectomorph has a long and lean shape with slender and delicate features, is restrained, tense, sensitive, prefers solitude, and is likely to have allergies.

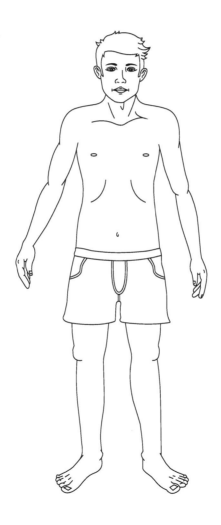

ECTOMORPH

Mesomorph

The mesomorph has a square shape with a firm body, rugged muscles, is active, energetic, noisy and assertive in temperament.

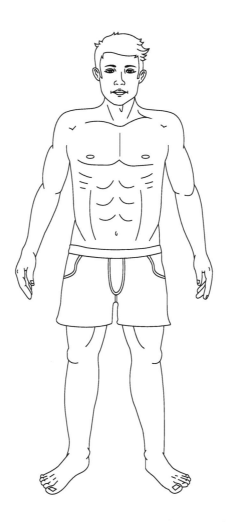

MESOMORPH

Endomorph

The endomorph has a round shape with a soft body, short neck, small hands and feet, experiences good digestion, is social, communicative and good-natured.

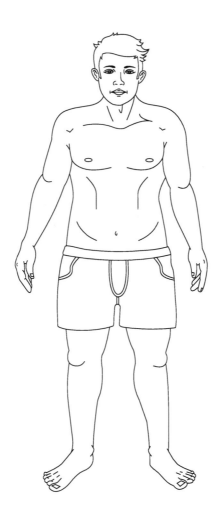

ENDOMORPH

Individuals are usually a combination of the body types, such as a mesomorphic ectomorph, that is, a strong, muscular but lean build, or a mesomorphic endomorph, which translates as a strong, muscular "hefty" build. Understanding your body type can help identify which sports would most suit you, increasing your chances of consistently participating, and staying healthy as a result.

Unlike its Western counterpart, fitness, according to ancient Chinese tradition, has always incorporated the body, mind and spirit. Exercise in Chinese philosophy and medicine is needed to achieve a state of health and harmony, and is designed to last a lifetime. If the body's energy or qi is balanced throughout the body, then the person is healthy. Two types of Chinese exercise specifically developed for obtaining optimum health are qi gong and taiqi chuan.

The word qigong has meaning: "qi" refers to the life force or energy in our body, and "gong" refers to effort or work. Qi gong is characterized by slow and gentle movements requiring mental focus. The breathing is natural and from the abdomen or "lower dan tian" area. The dan tian supports your body while it moves, and aids in moving the energy throughout the body. In qi gong, the tongue is placed on the roof of the mouth, to connect the energy from the front and back of the body. This body and mind collaboration, consistent with Chinese exercise ideals, harmonizes the body, balances the emotions and soothes the spirit.

The origin of this energy work dates back to the time of Fu Xi and is discussed in the *Book of Changes,* or *I Ching*. The movements were intended to relieve the damp diseases, such as arthritis, muscle ailments and skin diseases that plagued people living in harsh and cold climates during that time. Around 600 BCE, the physician Bien Que in the *Nan Jing*, mentioned specific breathing techniques to increase qi circulation. Approximately 200 CE, during the Han dynasty, drawings of forty qigong postures were circulated. Around 500 CE, a Buddhist monk named Da Mao went to the Shaolin Temple and, while living there for many years, wrote *Muscle/Tendon Changing Classic* or *Yi Jin Jing* and *Marrow/Brain Washing Classic* or *Xi Sui Jing*. These books explained how qigong would strengthen the blood, immune system and brain, helping the monks not just to recover from sickness but to achieve the type of optimal health needed to attain their goal of true enlightenment. In 1954, the first qigong convalescent hospital opened in Tangshan, in Hebei province, China. Currently, qigong is the subject of many ongoing medical research projects.

There are five major styles of qigong. The Taoist style is focused on self-cultivation. The Buddhist style emphasizes freeing the mind and achieving enlightenment. Confucian qigong is practiced to increase moral character and intelligence. Martial arts qigong stresses physical development, protecting the body from attack and directing qi to deliver traumatic blows. Lastly, medical qigong focuses on removing qi stagnations and blockages, and promoting the free flow of qi to relieve illness and injury.

Taiji chuan is the other Chinese exercise that promotes whole body health. Like qigong, taiji chuan has a specific meaning: "taiji" is translated as "grand ultimate" and chuan is translated as "fist," so taiji chuan is understood to mean the "grand ultimate fist." It is also referred to as shadow boxing. When travelling by bus to Chenjiagou, in the Henan province of China, one passes a massive stone sculpture of a single big fist, a famous landmark that lets every traveller know that they have arrived in taiji chuan country. This internal martial art incorporates the yin-yang principle in its exercise regimen. The moves are hard and soft, open and closed, light and heavy, fast and slow and up and down. Historically, taiji chuan was used to fight and so emphasized strength, balance, flexibility, speed and a strong mind as counters to brute force. Currently, taiji chuan has evolved into more of a gentle, slow, light form of exercise, one easily used by practitioners of all ages.

The *Book of Changes*, or *I Ching,* mentions taiji chuan along with qigong. Zhang Sanfeng, a legendary Daoist sage, was supposedly the individual who developed taiji chuan. This martial art was originally a combination of daoist philosophy and boxing, thought of as an "internal" school of boxing. During the Han Dynasty, scholars mentioned how taiji chuan encompassed the yin-yang principles of male and female, moon and sun, day and night, inhaling and exhaling and soft and hard. The first written record of taiji chuan begins around 1644 from the Chen family, in particular Chen Wangting, in the Chen village of Chenjiagou, China. This is the birthplace of taiji chuan. Chen Wangting was a Ming Dynasty officer, warrior and scholar. He wanted to train other warriors internally and externally. He taught one form that was soft, had varying speeds and was very powerful, and a second form that was hard and fast.

Five generations later, Chen Changxing taught Chen taiji to an outsider named Yang Luchan. He eventually formulated his own style called Yang taiji. To this day, this remains a popular taiji chuan style. At the beginning of the twentieth century, the great grandson of Chen Changxing, Chen Fake, started teaching classes in Bejing to the public. There are five taiji styles today: the Chen style, the Yang style, the Wu style, the Hao style, and the Sun style.

The Chen style has a special feature known as silk-reeling force, or *chansi jin*. With silk-reeling, there is a circular, spiral pattern to the smooth movements. Once the silk-reeling technique has been mastered, an explosive and powerful energy, or *fa-jing,* can occur. The Yang style has slow, flowing, expansive movements. The Wu style has gentle, slow movements that are tight and compact, with leaning postures. The Hao style has small, compact movements with upright postures. The Sun style has tight and compact movements with a high stance and fast pace.

(As a side note, in March of 2011 I visited Chenjiagou, China to study Chen taiji chuan under the instruction of Grandmaster Chen Xiaowang. The experience was amazing and powerful. Hundreds of people from all over the world came to attend this one week seminar for taiji chuan training. The qi circulating was astounding. I realized after attending this seminar that the only way to truly understand taiji chuan is to practice it consistently. I am only at the beginning of this internal martial art journey, but I look forward to trying to master its unique soft and hard, slow and fast, yin-yang qualities. Even for a novice like myself with a lifetime more to learn and experience, I felt great peace after the training, for me a very personal testament to its transformative power.)

There are also five body type classifications in Chinese philosophy and medicine, built around the five elements of wood, fire, earth, metal, water.

Illustrations for each of these five body types follow.

Wood Type

The wood type individual has a muscular and square physique with thick skin and strong hands. This athlete loves action, adventure, seeks a challenge, can push to the limit and does well under pressure. One would find plenty of examples of wood types at a decathlon or eco-challenge.

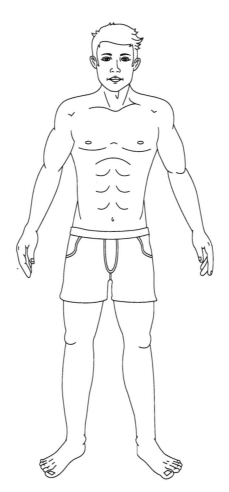

WOOD TYPE

Fire Type

The fire type individual has a soft and willowy physique, long neck and limbs, soft skin and graceful hands. This type loves excitement and drama, and is charismatic and focused. Any performance sport like dance or musical theater would be ideal for this body type.

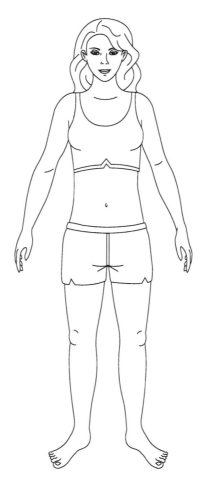

FIRE TYPE

Earth Type

The earth type individual has a round and firm body with large and thick muscles. The hands and feet seem small and the skin is soft and smooth. This type of athlete is easy-going and likes to be part of a team. Baseball, football, soccer, basketball or other team sports would be suitable for an earth type.

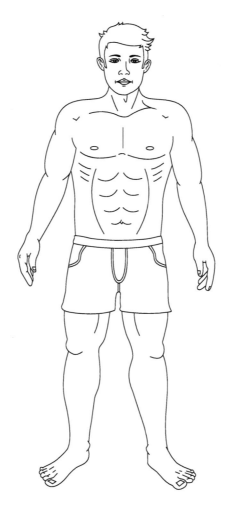

EARTH TYPE

Metal Type

The metal type athlete has a trim and symmetrical physique with compact muscles, small bones and clear skin. This type enjoys discipline, precision and admires art, so ballet, archery or fencing would be appropriate sport choices.

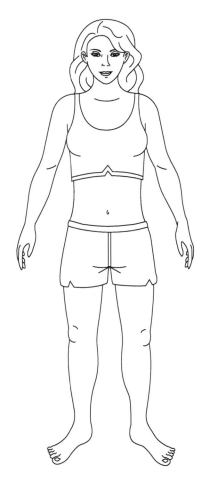

METAL TYPE

Water Type

The water type individual has a dense, lean and strong body. This type has a sculptured face and deep-set eyes. This athlete is introspective, sensible and curious, so hiking and kayaking would be appropriate sports.

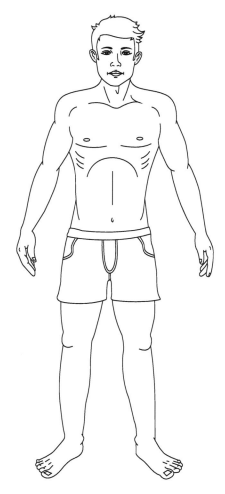

WATER TYPE

Having looked at both the Western and Chinese approaches to exercise, and viewed examples of each of their body types, let's move on to Ayurvedic philosophy and medicine. Similar to the Chinese fitness philosophy, it promotes physical activity so that the whole person - the body, mind and spirit - can be healthy. Yoga is the exercise regimen most closely associated with the Ayurvedic tradition. It means "union," and not just in the Western sense of bringing together body and mind, but also of connecting with God. This spiritual emphasis is an intrinsic and valuable aspect of yoga.

The oldest written book, the *Rig Veda*, mentions yoga. The *Rig Veda's* lessons about yoga were taught by Hindu sages. Around 600 BCE, Buddhism added to yoga practice, emphasizing meditation along with the execution of special physical postures. Approximately 200 CE, a scholar named Patanjali wrote the *Eight Limbs of Classical Yoga*, or *Yoga Sutra*, to standardize classical yoga. Patanjali discussed ethics or *yama*, purity or *niyama*, physical exercise or *asanas*, breathing or *pranayama*, preparation for meditation or *pratahara*, concentration or *dharana*, meditation or *dhyana*, and deep mediation or *samadhi*. Around the mid-1800's, Western culture began to embrace yoga. By the 1930's, practicing yoga exercise and eating a vegetarian diet continued to grow in popularity in the West. By the 1960's, yoga masters from India were travelling to America to personally spread their practice. During this time, Maharishi Mahesh popularized Transcendental Meditation, and Swami Sivananda opened yoga schools and authored hundreds of books about yoga and its philosophy. Recently, according to the National Sporting Goods Association's Annual 2010 Sports Participation report, U.S. participation in yoga has sky-rocketed. Yoga has increased 28.1% to 20.2 million participants, the largest single-year-increase registered for any "sport."

There are many styles of yoga, with the most popular being Hatha, Vinyasa, Ashtanga, Iyengar and Bikram. Hatha yoga has gentle, slow movements and postures with breathing techniques.

Vinyasa yoga has vigorous movement with breathing that coordinates with each movement. Ashtanga yoga is a powerful, aerobic and fast moving yoga. Iyengar yoga focuses on moving with the correct body alignment. Bikram yoga is practiced in a heated room for detoxification and to prevent injuries.

Yoga describes specific breathing techniques and postures that are designed to affect the doshas, regulate temperature and stimulate or calm the body. Some examples include inhaling with the left nostril and exhaling with the right nostril in order to calm the body; inhaling through a curled tongue and exhaling with a left nostril in order to cool the body; inhaling with the right nostril and exhaling with left nostril to stimulate the body; and rapidly inhaling through both nostrils and then rapidly exhaling through both nostrils in order to induce a heating effect on the body. In addition, inhaling with the left nostril, exhaling with the right nostril, and then inhaling with the right nostril and exhaling with the left nostril, attempts to balance vata, pitta and kapha. For the postures, inhaling and back-bending movements support kapha, while exhaling and forward bending, twisting movements, or inverted poses, support vata and pitta.

Breathing

Calming   *Inhale left nostril; exhale right nostril*

Cooling   *Inhale through curled tongue; exhale left nostril*

Balancing   *Inhale left nostril; exhale right nostril; inhale right nostril; exhale left nostril*

Stimulating   *Inhale right nostril; exhale left nostril*

Heating   *Rapid inhale both nostrils; rapid exhale both nostrils*

Postures

Vatta and Pitta

Exhaling

Forward bends

Twisting

Inverted poses

Kapha

Inhaling

Back-bending movement

Ayurvedic exercise also has body typing, like Western and Chinese exercise. It describes the types according to the vata, pitta and kapha doshas.

Illustrations for each of these three body types follow.

Vata Body Type

The vata body type has a lean and thin muscle physique with quick metabolism. Vata types will excel in sports requiring quick bursts of speed and agility. This type is similar to thoroughbred race horses, so they can become very restless, even jumpy at times. Too much fast, vigorous activity can cause imbalance for a vata type, so cross-training is suggested with moderate amounts of low-impact, medium-intensity exercise. Vata types prefer racquetball, ping-pong, sprinting, gymnastics, aerobics, dance, in particular, ballet. To keep in balance, they also need to include low-impact jogging, walking, cycling, swimming, hiking or yoga.

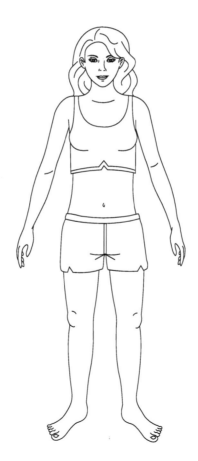

VATA BODY TYPE

Pitta Body Type

The pitta body type has defined muscles throughout their physique. The pitta body type is successful in sport competitions requiring strength, speed and stamina. This type is highly motivated, driven and wants to win. To balance their fierce competitive nature, this type needs to enjoy non-competitive sports and find activities that are cooling in nature. The pitta types prefer rock climbing, martial arts, skydiving, weightlifting and competitive tennis, track and field, ice skating, downhill skiing, surfing, and swimming. To balance their body, the pitta type needs to also engage in activities like cross-country skiing, racquet sports, cycling, golf, recreational swimming and body surfing.

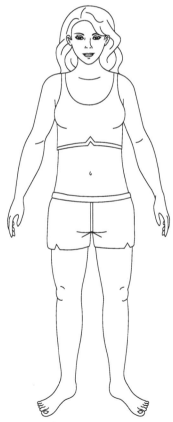

PITTA BODY TYPE

Kapha Body Type

A kapha body type has a large, fleshy physique. The kapha type does well with endurance sports requiring a lot mental focus such as hitting a baseball or shooting an arrow. The kapha type has a calm and easy-going disposition and is great under pressure. Sometimes, a kapha type becomes unmotivated to exercise, so vigorous aerobic exercise to stay balanced and help the metabolism is required. A kapha type prefers baseball, football, hockey, archery, golf, cycling, hiking, horseback riding but also needs active sports such as tennis, racquetball, rowing, running, swimming, shaping up boot camps, aerobics or gymnastics.

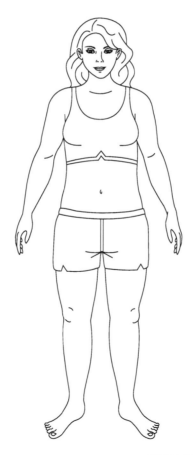

KAPHA BODY TYPE

The Western, Chinese and Ayruvedic exercise traditions all emphasize the necessity of physical activity for proper health; in addition, they all have body types and all consider breathing a vital aspect of exercise. Breathing is also a common focus: aerobic movement is key for effective Western exercise, Chinese exercise focuses on breathing from the dan tian to cultivate good energy, and yoga has specific breathing techniques to optimize each position.

The first principle of my own "cross-cultural" fitness program, *Exaircise*, draws on this common focus, and begins by emphasizing breathing. We actually must first "remember" how to fully inhale and exhale naturally. There are two types of breathing, diaphragmatic and chest breathing. Diaphragmatic breathing has slow and rhythmic inhalations and exhalations with large volumes of air exchanged. A diaphragmatic type of breather has a lower heart rate, and decreased cardio-pulmonary stress, muscle tension, perception of pain and need for sleep. The diaphragmatic breather also has emotional stability and confidence. Chest breathing, or thoracic breathing, has rapid and irregular inhalations and exhalations with low volumes of air exchanged. A chest breather has a rising heart rate, and increased cardio-pulmonary stress, muscle tension, perception of pain and need for sleep. The chest breather has decreased emotional stability with increased fearfulness, shyness and anxiety.

Diaphragmatic

Low heart rate

Decreased cardio-pulmonary stress

Decreased muscle tension

Decreased perception of pain

Decreased need for sleep

Emotional stability and confidence

Thoracic

Rising heart rate

Increased cardio-pilmonary stress

Increased muscle tension

Increased perception of pain

Increased need for sleep

Increased fearfulness

Shyness and anxiety

While explaining the *Exaircise* philosophy, I will share stories from clients I trained. Their success stories will help support the importance of exercising properly. The first of these is from one of my clients, Sally, who had tried every diet and every fitness craze to lose weight. I watched her body movement and explained that I noticed she wasn't breathing properly. We reviewed the natural or belly breathing technique along with some gentle, floor exercises as an exercise program. Within three weeks, working out two times a week for one hour, Sally lost two dress sizes, moving down from a size 14 to a 10. She was very pleased and surprised what a difference efficient breathing could make. Not only did she lose inches but she also discovered how enjoyable exercise and movement can be.

The second principle of the *Exaircise* approach involves movement awareness. Tai qi, qi gong, and yoga all emphasize an awareness of body movement while practicing their particular exercise techniques: tai qi and qi gong with slow movements, and yoga with verbal instruction from the teacher to help students notice how strained or easily they are moving during training. The result is that the body stops moving as a collection of rigid segments and begins having its independent body parts move as one in a fluid and flexible manner. Additionally, what really facilitates the incredible experience of true muscle sensory awareness, is the incorporation of proper breathing, as described in the first principle, into exercise movement. The air will help you feel how to move lightly but still have power, and the movement awareness will assist in how to move correctly and fluidly, not tensely intertwined. For example, when you are moving your arms, does your neck tighten, do your shoulders rise up to your ears, does your back arch and your belly hang out? All that stress and misalignment can cause injury to your body. It is important to just feel your arm move while your neck relaxes, your shoulders stay down, your back feels like it's lengthening and your belly "informs" the whole movement with your breath. In this way, the arm exercise will be properly supported and the energy flow and power will increase. As you exercise, you can feel your whole body move and support the specific area that you are working to its greatest potential. Using this technique is crucial in preventing injury while exercising. With this particular example – developing muscle awareness about arm movement - headaches, neck tightness and pinched nerves will be prevented.

Another area that holds a lot of tension are the hips. If the hips are tight, diets and hip exercises won't entirely change their shape. In order for any change to take place, the circulation must flow and the hips and low back must relax, so that the belly breathing can support the exercise. The first step is to notice the hip tension and the second step is to incorporate the proper breathing into an appropriate exercise. When these two processes are in action together, the desired bodyshaping can result. John was athletic. He liked rock climbing, weightlifting and cycling. To increase his flexibility, movement awareness and cardiovascular stamina, we reviewed the way he moved his lower body. We discovered his overdeveloped quadriceps created an imbalance. He needed to feel his hamstrings move more effectively and he needed to loosen up his lower back. By changing his concentration to the back of his body and by using simple and effective isolated muscle awareness exercises, his stamina and flexibility increased. He even started to place in his cycling races.

The third principle of the *Exaircise* program entails alignment focus. This concept creates better balance and safety for your body, and not just when you are exercising. Chinese exercise accomplishes this by having tai qi use soft and hard movements to convey being grounded, centered and body balanced, while Ayurvedic exercise has yoga using specific flexibility and strengthening techniques to develop proper alignment and balance. An example of alignment focus, using the *Exaircise* methodology, is when your right leg is kicking up toward the sky, the left leg must be pressing into the floor to give the body the balance needed to support the right leg height. The alignment of the left leg is just as important as action of the right leg. There must be push (into the ground) and pull (into the air) energy working at all times for correct balance. This concept is subtle and requires mental focus but is essential for successful exercise. This example also shows how the right and left side of the body must work together to provide proper movement.

Using all three *Exaircise* concepts - breathing, movement awareness and alignment focus - will make a body vital, strong and flexible. One final, real-life example: Bill was preparing for a taekwondo tournament to perform a forms routine. Bill had power but needed more flexibility when kicking in his form. When he would do a side kick, he would only think about the kicking leg. Only when he was taught how to push the supporting non-kicking leg firmly into the ground and lift up his upper body, could he then pull the side kicking leg up higher. He now had a flexible and powerful side kick. He received higher scores in his forms performance and placed in the top three during the tournament.

Another example of how the upper and lower body must use alignment focus is during running. Moving and pumping your legs is necessary but we now know that pumping your arms is also important. As the lower body is working, the upper body must not be slouching but rather pumping its arms while supporting and balancing the pumping of the legs. The next time you are running, notice when your legs are tired and if your arms are at that point helping with the overall movement and themselves pumping. If the arms are tight, try to relax and use your breath to help them pump and move, then notice the resurgence of energy in your lower body, and see if you are capable of running further.

In 2001, according to the *New England Journal of Medicine,* about two-thirds of adults have experienced low back pain at some time in their lives. Since back pain is quite common, it is a good place to leverage the benefits of alignment focus on the front and back of the body. Many times the back is tight and needs to let go of the aggravating tension. If the body is supported with proper breathing from the abdomen and diaphragm, if the muscle awareness of the rigid back can relax while the powerful abdomen does the support and work, if the front and back of the body are effectively working together, and, finally, if the feeling of the alignment of the spine is long and light, the conditions have been created for the back pain to subside. Proper breathing, muscle awareness and alignment focus are powerful techniques that allow for not just a healthy back, but a healthy, vibrant body.

So far, though we have used both general and real-life examples, our overview of the *Exaircise* program has been on a conceptual basis. In keeping with one of the goals of this book, to not just provide an overview of the three main medical modalities but to also illustrate each main topic with useful, interactive exercises, what follows is a practical guide to some of the *Exaircise* program's more important routines. Many of these routines will reinforce the conceptual principles we've just introduced.

Exaircise is a simple movement program for all ages. The exercises begin with reminding our body how to "belly breathe." To get back-to-the-basics, and remind our bodies how to breath naturally, first lie down on the floor or on a comfortable flat surface. Make certain that your back is flat and your chin is down. Place one hand on your belly button and one hand on your sternum or chest bone. Begin simply inhaling as much air as you possibly can. Balloon your belly. Be sure that not only your rib cage space is full of air, but the space around your belly button is expanding as well. After you have filled up with as much air as possible, slowly deflate your abdomen and chest area and begin to exhale. Make sure that your back stays flat to the floor throughout this process. Repeat this pattern for five times.

To get even more comfortable with this technique, try the following exercise. Not only will you perfect this important breathing style but you will also start to flatten your tummy. As always, lie down on a flat surface and check your back and chin for proper alignment. Slowly inhale; in fact, take four counts to inhale. Now, hold that inhale for four counts. Next, exhale slowly for four counts. Lastly, keep your body empty without any air for four counts. Repeat this exercise five times. Once this feels comfortable, increase each step of the exercise to eight and then twelve counts. Feel the belly power.

Once lying down feels comfortable, try this exercise sitting up and finally, try this exercise standing. This is ideally the way you want to breathe 24 hours a day.

Remembering the three key concepts of *Exaircise* – proper breathing, muscle awareness and alignment focus, let's move on to more challenging routines. These exercises will help you feel the connection of your breath with your movement, elongate and release stress from your back and hamstrings, open up your hip area and energize your body.

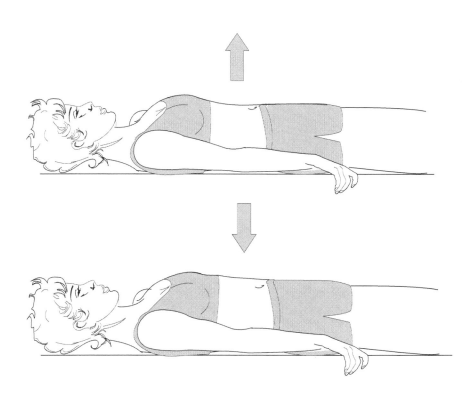

Sacrum Tilting

This exercise will help to relax the base of your spine or sacrum.
Lie on your back and bend your knees. Cross your arms over your
chest. Keep your neck long and chin in. Inhale and don't move.
Next, as you exhale, ever so gently tilt your tailbone up and down.
Picture your triangular-shaped sacrum rocking up and down in
small movements. This is a small motion but very important in
releasing back tension. Repeat five times.

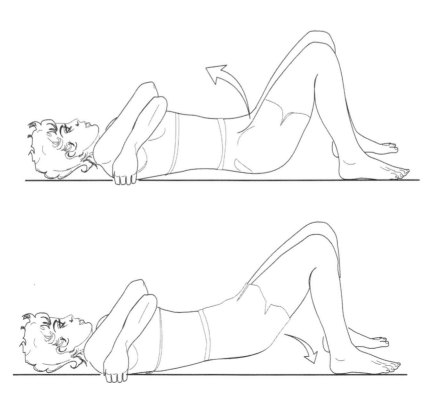

The Shaker

This exercise will help your body relax from the sacrum to your toes. Lie on your back and bend knees. Keep your neck long and chin in. There are three parts to this exercise. First, inhale and bring one knee to your chest. Use your hands to support your hamstring muscles. Second, start to exhale and flex your foot. Third, still exhaling, extend your heel up and find the place where your leg and thigh start to shake naturally. The more natural the shaking, the better it is for your back and hamstrings. Shake for 10 seconds or until your leg stops moving. It isn't necessary to have your leg straight, if it naturally straightens, then fine. In the beginning, you may only feel the shaking in the calf. It will work its way from the calf, down the thigh and then into the sacrum area. Feel the supporting bent leg press firmly into the ground. Keep your hip area flat on the floor. This movement will relax your lower body. Do this exercise three times and then change sides.

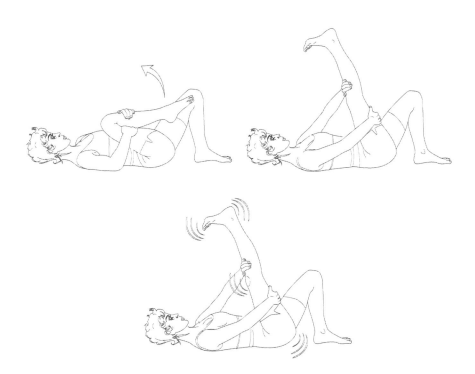

Drag Swings

This exercise will help to lengthen your hamstrings. Lie flat on your back and bend your knees. Keep your arms crossed over your chest, neck long and chin in. Inhale and bend one knee up toward your chest. As you move that knee away from your chest, exhale and drag the foot on the ground as long as possible until you feel that you can gently spring your leg up in the air. Do not lift your leg up in the air. Reverse your movement direction to complete the exercise. Lifting makes your leg feel heavy and springing makes your leg feel light. The other bent leg has its hip area and foot pressing firmly into the ground. Do this five times and then change sides.

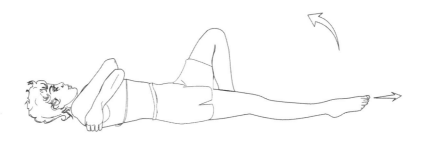

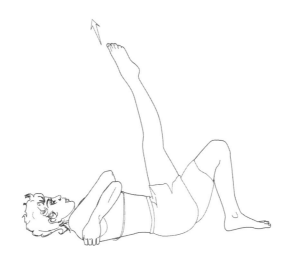

Adductor Squeeze

This exercise will make you more aware of your inner thighs. Lie on your back, neck long and chin in. Bring knees up toward your chest and open laterally. Make certain your heels are higher than your knees. Place your hands on the inner thighs. Inhale and don't move. Exhale as you press your knees closer to the mid line of your body. Resist with your hands as you press in. Create as little or as much tension as you need. Feel the inner thighs working. Keep exhaling as you return the original position. Repeat 10 times.

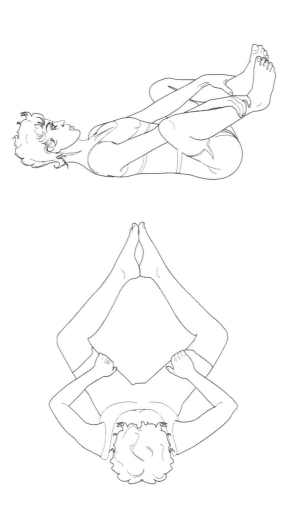

Hip Turns

This exercise will make you aware of your range of motion in the abductor or hip area. Lie on your back with knees bent, neck long and chin in. Raise one leg toward your chest with the knee relaxed. Place the hand on the same side of your body on the inner thigh to gently support that raised leg. Feel the other leg and thigh pressed firmly into the floor surface. Inhale and don't move then exhale and let your raised leg rotate laterally. Inhale as you return to the original position. Feel how much that hip can easily rotate. Do five times then change to the other side.

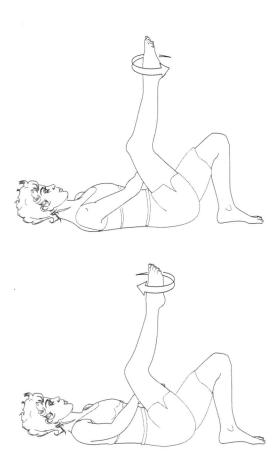

Side Swings

This exercise will help you loosen up the hip area. Lie on one side of your body. Cradle your head on the arm closest to the floor. The other arm helps to support your sideways position. Bend your knees up toward your chest with the leg closest to the floor curled up more than the other leg. Take the leg furthest from the floor and with its toe, draw a half circle. Inhale and start curving to the back of your body and then exhale as the toe moves toward your chest while circling around your other leg. Make certain your hip stays facing toward the front of your body. Don't let your hip area open up sideways. Return to the original forward position. Do five times then change to the other side.

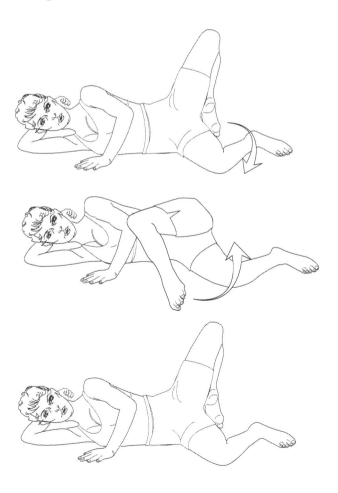

There are many people who just don't make the time to exercise. The following exercises are for just those people. These exercises can be done at your desk while working, or in a chair while watching television. These exercises are recommended to be done daily and designed to energize. It is a much healthier way to relieve stress and rejuvenate your body than drinking coffee or snacking on candy bars.

Desk Exaircises

Belly Breathing   *Do five times.*

Extended Breathing   *Using the Belly Breathing technique, inhale for four counts, hold the air for four counts, exhale for four counts and be empty without air for four counts. Do the extended breathing two times.*

Shoulder Shrugs   *Inhale before moving, then exhale as you pull your shoulders up to your ears and lower to original position. Do shoulder shrugs five times.*

Shoulder Rolls   *Inhale before moving then exhale as you roll your shoulders toward the back of your body five times.*

Chin retractions   *Pull your chin in to your neck. Inhale and don't move. Exhale as you move back to your original position. Do chin retractions two times.*

Wrist Flicks   *Inhale before moving then exhale while you flap your hands up and down loosely ten times. Next, inhale before moving then exhale as you flap your hands side to side* *for 10 repetitions. Feel the circulation in your wrists.*

Pelvic Tilts   *Inhale and don't move. As you exhale, gently rock tailbone up and down. Do pelvic tilts five times.*

Inner Thigh Squeezes   *Inhale and notice the inside of your thighs. As you exhale, press your inner thighs against the air. Create as little or as much tension when pressing to notice your inner thigh area. Repeat squeezes five times.*

Outer Thigh Squeezes   *Inhale and notice the outside thigh area. As you exhale, press your thighs against the air. Create as little or as much tension while noticing the outside thigh area. Repeat squeezes five times.*

Ankle Circles   *Inhale and lift one foot. Exhale as you circle clockwise five times. Inhale again and lift the same foot. Exhale as you circle counter-clockwise five times. Repeat on other foot. Feel the circulation in the ankles.*

Taking care of your body is of utmost importance. The theme for a strong mind is to have a strong body. Make sure you are breathing and breathing correctly, be aware of how you are moving and make certain you are not just "going through the motions" of movement and exercise, and notice your proper alignment when moving through your day so your body doesn't become injured or so stressed. Be vital and happy. At **vitalityfusion.com,** you can download additional body charts, a measurement chart and an exercise awareness chart. The following body charts identify basic muscles you use everyday. The body measurement chart is for your reference. Keep track of how your shape positively changes as you *Exaircise* your way to health. Also, notice how you feel when you exercise. What are your thoughts during exercise? What parts of your body do you feel the most during exercise? This awareness will give insight on how focused and connected you are to your body, and what areas may need attention and realignment to be properly exercised. Your thoughts, feelings and mindfulness while exercising are interconnected with your body successfully training and achieving strength, flexibility and overall well-being. The next chapter will further explore how the mind and body are intertwined. This chapter discussed how powerful and healthy the body can be and the next chapter will elaborate how the mind can increase the vitality of the body if they work together in harmony.

Body Measurement Chart

Before you begin shaping up, measure yourself. Periodically, measure again and see your positive progress.
Fill out the measurements for:

Body Part	Inches/Date	Inches/Date	Inches/Date
UPPER ARM			
CHEST			
WAIST			
HIPS			
THIGHS			

Clothing Sizes	Size/Date	Size/Date	Size/Date
DRESS OR SUIT			
SKIRT OR PANTS			
BLOUSE OR SHIRT			
SWIM ATTIRE			

Muscle Chart Front of Body

PECTORALIS MAJOR
AND MINOR

BICEPS BRACHII

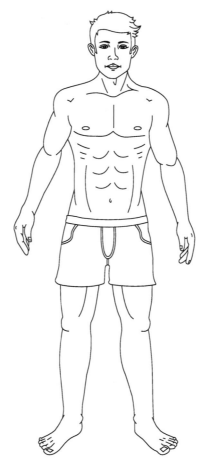

ABDOMEN:

RECTUS ABDOMINIS

TRANSVERSUS ABDOMINIS

EXTERNAL OBLIQUES

INTERNAL OBLIQUES

QUADRICEPS FEMORIS:
RECTUS FEMORIS
VASTUS MEDIALIS
VASTUS LATERALIS
VASTUS INTERMEDIUS

ADDUCTORS:

ADDUCTOR BREVIS

ADDUCTOR LONGUS

ADDUCTOR MAGNUS

GRACILIS

LEG / TIBIALIS ANTERIOR

Muscle Chart Back of Body

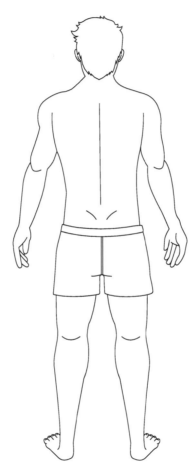

SHOULDER / DELTOID

TRICEPS BRACHII

HAMSTRINGS:
BICEPS FEMORIS
SEMITENDINOSUS
SEMIMEMBRANOSUS

CALF / SOLEUS
AND GASTROCNEMIUS

UPPER AND MIDDLE BACK:
TRAPEZIUS
LEVATOR SCAPULAE
TERES MAJOR
RHOMBOIDS
LATISSIMUS DORSI

ABDUCTORS:
GLUTEUS MAXIMUS
GLUTEUS MEDIUS
GLUTEUS MINIMUS

LEG / PERONEUS LONGUS
AND PERONEUS BREVIS

Body Awareness Diary

Date	Type of exercise	Feelings and thoughts During Exercise	Body awareness notes
	swimming	I am happy and feel strong when in the water.	My right leg kicks harder than my left leg ; my neck turns easily to the right.

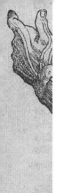

Chapter Six:
Mind Body Connection

"What your minds dwells upon, the body acts upon."
- DENIS WAITLEY

Understanding that Chinese and Ayurvedic medicine have always considered the mental, emotional and physical aspects of a body to be interconnected, and realizing that there has been a growing realization and confirmation of this link in Western medicine, all three healthcare modalities are now on common ground regarding the mind body connection. A Harvard researcher, Dr. Herbert Benson, explored the traditions of the East while visiting the Himalayas around 30 years ago. He filmed a practice of the Buddhist monks there, in which they wrapped themselves in icy sheets, in a 40-degree Fahrenheit (or 4.4 degree Celsius) room, and through their ability to regulate their own body temperature, made the sheets steam within three minutes. They completely dried the sheets within 30 minutes. Another amazing example of the mind body connection observed by Dr. Benson was watching the monks on a 19,000 foot precipice, in zero degree weather, wearing nothing but a thin cotton shawl, and walking through the snow in sandals without socks. They generated heat from their yoga and advanced meditative processes. The power of the mind over the body as recorded in these examples is equally astounding.

Dr. Benson is now considered the "father of mind body medicine" and was a founder of the Benson-Henry Institute for Mind Body Medicine in Massachusetts. In 1974, Dr. Benson defined the relaxation response when he discovered there was an opposite state to the stress response, or the fight and flight response. The relaxation response is a physical state of deep rest that changes the physical and emotional responses to stress. Methods that encourage the development of the relaxation response include meditation, mindfulness, progressive muscle relaxation, tai chi and yoga. These techniques help the body to lower blood pressure and heart rate, decrease rapid breathing and lessen muscle tension.

The relaxation and stress responses are intertwined within our nervous system. The relaxation response is a part of our parasympathetic system and our stress response is a part of our sympathetic system. These two systems are a part of the autonomic section of the peripheral nervous system. The somatic section, which controls skeletal muscles, is also a part of the peripheral nervous system. The central nervous system communicates with the brain and spinal cord. Both the peripheral nervous system and central nervous system make up the nervous system. The chart below illustrates this relationship.

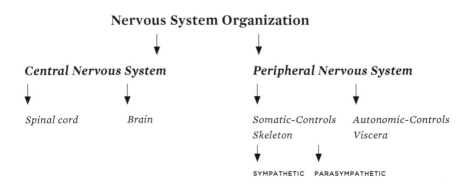

Nervous System Organization

Central Nervous System

Spinal cord   *Brain*

Peripheral Nervous System

Somatic-Controls Skeleton   *Autonomic-Controls Viscera*

SYMPATHETIC   PARASYMPATHETIC

This nervous system physiology helps to explain how our body and mind are inseparable. Another way to appreciate the body and mind connection is to look at our everyday life: if you mentally or emotionally had a rough day at the office, and ended up arguing with your boss or colleague, you might develop a headache or neck tension later in the day. If you physically trained extra hard for an upcoming triathlon during the day, later in the evening you might feel so exhausted and fatigued that you can't think clearly and become indecisive. If you had a beautiful relaxing day at the beach, your body might "smile" and feel light while you feel imbued with a happy afterglow. These upsetting or wonderful feelings and emotions come from the mind and send tense or relaxed responses throughout your body. Studies are continually confirming the benefits of a relaxed response, and the health detriments of sustained stress.

There are many techniques that work with the body and mind to relieve physical, mental and emotional stress while encouraging ways to live a more joyful life. From a structural body perspective, in the 1940's, Dr. Ida Rolf, a biochemist, began applying her structural integration program with clients. Gravity affected the body, its proper alignment and overall sense of well-being. Imbalances in the structure caused problems for the muscles, fascia, tendons and ligaments. This disruption caused illness and lack of well-being. Ida Rolf developed a program with ten sessions to correct the structure. Dr. Joseph Heller studied with Ida Rolf. In the 1970's, he developed his own program, Hellerwork Structural Integration. This program has eleven sessions of deep-tissue structural integration bodywork, dialogue about emotions and movement education. The movement education allows for long lasting effects from the bodywork and dialogue sessions.

From a psychological perspective, in the 1950's, Bioenergetics, primarily founded by Dr. Alexander Lowen, with the help of John Pierrakos and William Waller, both psychiatrists, looked at muscle tensions and contracted postures to help identify energy and emotional blockages, or armoring, in the body. Bioenergetic exercises were taught to release pain and infuse confidence and a sense of well-being.

In 1977, Ken Dychtwald, a psychologist who studied with Dr. Lowen and John Pierrakos, published *Bodymind*. This book looks at what emotion is stored in what body part. Some examples of the body areas and the corresponding emotions are that feet represent stability and feeling emotionally grounded, legs support and carry the body and create a sense of security, ankles and knees help the body move and flow and support physical, mental and emotional transitions the body experiences. Moving up the body, the abdomen is the feeling center of our body, where emotions are created. The low back reflects how controlling or impulsively the body flows through everyday life. For example, a tight back indicates a person with a structured daily schedule while a flexible back signifies a person without much plan or is quite spontaneous. The middle and upper back represent feelings of responsibility and guilt. The chest and diaphragm are where feelings are processed and then sent through the arms to be expressed, with the elbows helping the emotions to transition and move through the body. The heart amplifies our feelings in a loving and affectionate manner. The neck translates and refines our communication of feelings into thoughts and words. In this system, the head represents the image the world gets to see and protects or displays emotions inside the body.

Front Mind Body Chart

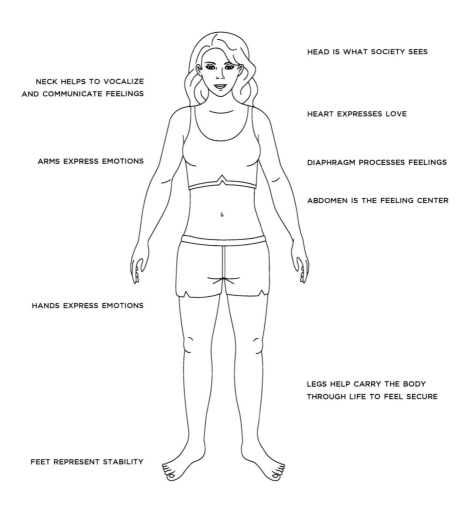

HEAD IS WHAT SOCIETY SEES

NECK HELPS TO VOCALIZE
AND COMMUNICATE FEELINGS

HEART EXPRESSES LOVE

ARMS EXPRESS EMOTIONS

DIAPHRAGM PROCESSES FEELINGS

ABDOMEN IS THE FEELING CENTER

HANDS EXPRESS EMOTIONS

LEGS HELP CARRY THE BODY
THROUGH LIFE TO FEEL SECURE

FEET REPRESENT STABILITY

Back Mind Body Chart

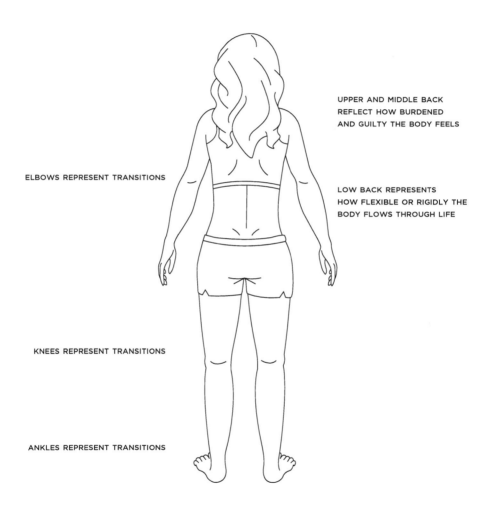

UPPER AND MIDDLE BACK
REFLECT HOW BURDENED
AND GUILTY THE BODY FEELS

ELBOWS REPRESENT TRANSITIONS

LOW BACK REPRESENTS
HOW FLEXIBLE OR RIGIDLY THE
BODY FLOWS THROUGH LIFE

KNEES REPRESENT TRANSITIONS

ANKLES REPRESENT TRANSITIONS

Another system views the body according to "body splits." The five body splits are right and left, top and bottom, front and back, torso and limbs and head and body. In particular, the right and left body split has become popular discussion among Western medical professionals. There has been a significant research focus on the right and left hemisphere of the brain, or the lateralization of brain function. In 1981, Roger Sperry, a physiological psychologist, received the Nobel Prize in medicine for his work regarding split brain research. During the 1950 and 60's, he and his colleagues discovered the special functions of the cerebral hemispheres. He was studying the effects of epilepsy, and discovered that cutting the corpus collosum could reduce or eliminate seizures. The corpus collosum is the nerve structure that connects the two hemispheres of the brain. After the cutting procedure, it was discovered that each hemisphere had specialized tasks. The left hemisphere takes care of language, analytical and critical thinking, numbers and logic. The right hemisphere takes care of recognizing faces, expressing and reading emotions, being creative and intuitive, recognizing color and playing music.

While Roger Sperry was absorbed analyzing the lateralization of brain function, an art therapist named Lucia Capacchione, Ph.D was equally engrossed in a bit of self-exploration, studying how she could use the right side of her own brain to heal and balance herself. The technique she developed involved handwriting, drawing and journaling. Her thinking was that since most people are right-handed, they therefore use the left side of their brain when handwriting. Writing with the left hand allows the right side of the brain to be engaged, and open up the body, creatively and intuitively. Lucia Capacchione went on to author many books, including *The Power of Your Other Hand*. In it, she discusses using both hands to write, draw and communicate, opening up a therapeutic and creative "dialogue" with the body. The dominant hand which you naturally write with and use the most, (in most cases, the right hand), and the non-dominant hand which is hardly used, (in most cases, the left hand), dialogue with each other to find out what the body needs to express. The dominant hand represents the adult thoughts and feelings in us, while the non-dominant hand represents the creative ideas and inner-child-playfulness in us.

I have personally written in journals most of my life. When I was younger, the journals had a little lock and tiny key. The journal was where I put my feelings, thoughts and animated figure drawings. It was a safe and fun place to record what I was experiencing without anyone else judging or commenting on my journey. When I was a young adult, I was curious and wanted to see what my inner child had to say. Was I taking good care of myself and listening to the playful and insightful side of myself? At the time, I was so busy working with fitness training clients and attending graduate school for Traditional Chinese Medicine, that I thought it was quite possible that I was neglecting my inner child. I decided to journal to my grown-up self with my dominant hand and my inner child with my non-dominant child. As I suspected, my inner child was tired from all the work and wanted to play. This insight was interesting but how could I add inner child play to my busy schedule? One idea came to mind. I set up a telephone joke hotline. My fitness clientele would use my confidential voice mail and leave jokes on the message machine. During fitness training appointments, I would share the jokes with various clients. We laughed so much during our training sessions, the playfulness added a special, wonderful dimension for not only me, but every one of my clients. The laughter was motivating and energizing: my clients would exercise, belly laugh and train even harder, with a lingering smile.

After graduate school, I worked in two offices as a licensed acupuncturist. I offered acupuncture, herbal medicine, nutrition counseling and my fitness exercises as elements of my treatment regimen. My working schedule consumed my day. My business was growing, and so was I, when I became pregnant with my first child. I loved my career so much that I worked up until the last week before my first child was born. It was during this immensely busy time that another idea occurred to me. Why not journal to not just to my adult self and my inner child, but also to the growing baby? Journaling to my baby, in utero, worked. I used my dominant hand to check-in with my grown-up self, my non-dominant hand to check-in with my inner child self, and then I used my non-dominant hand again to check-in with my growing baby.

Here is an excerpt from one of those pregnancy journal entries: With my dominant hand, I simply wrote the question, how are you baby? With my non-dominant hand, I quickly wrote the reply, "I am tired, I need more music- it is like food and water to me, I want to go to the park and I want more hugs." This let me know that I could play more music for my baby to listen to, I could rub my belly more to help hug my baby, and that I needed a walk in the park to rejuvenate myself and baby. I found the journaling easy to do and informative.

Reading to your baby is wonderful. Talking to your belly is fun. Rubbing your belly, as well as playing classical music, is soothing. When the baby arrives, I wish that a descriptive scroll about the baby would appear, some scroll that conveniently describes the child's strengths and interests, maybe even their life purpose. Since that scroll doesn't exist, baby journaling may be the next best way to connect and learn about your baby.

Visit **vitalityfusion.com** to print a copy of the journaling page which follows to give dominant and non-dominant handwriting a try. Use the dominant hand to ask any questions and use the non-dominant hand to write a reply or draw a picture. The question can be health-related, life purpose related, personal relationship related, and yes, even baby-on-the-way related. Let the creative and intuitive side of your brain speak and express the insight.

Journal Writing

The hand that you write with the most asks the question:

Why do I feel sad?

_____

_____

_____

_____

_____

_____

_____

_____

_____

_____

_____

_____

_____

With the hand you don't use for writing, write the reply:

I am tired and useless. I wish I had more time to play and
enjoy life. I want to make a difference in the world.

_____

_____

_____

_____

_____

_____

_____

_____

_____

_____

_____

_____

Dr. Joan Borysenko, biologist and licensed psychologist, worked with Dr. Herbert Benson during her third post-doctoral fellowship in psychoneuroimmunology, or PNI, and in the 1980's, and cofounded with Dr. Benson and Dr. Ilan Kutz, the Mind-Body Clinical Programs at the Beth Israel/Deaconess Medical Center in Boston. In Dr. Borysenko's book, *Minding the Body, Mending the Mind*, PNI describes and explains how you think determines how you feel, both physically and emotionally. When your thoughts create strong emotions, your brain releases hormones to communicate those emotions. These hormones are called neuropeptides. The neuropeptides get into the bloodstream and travel throughout the body. The neuropeptides manufactured by the immune system, or by different organs, can, conversely, affect the brain and emotional state.

The interconnectedness of the body and mind, their fundamental influence on each other, is quickly becoming a Western scientific reality. More and more studies arrive at the same conclusion – that a healthy body makes for a healthy mind, and that the mind exerts incredible power over the state of physical health. Western, Chinese and Ayurvedic medicine are in agreement about mind body connection. In the next chapter, let's explore some stress management options that each of the three modalities offer, and some preferred by Chinese and Ayurvedic practices that are valuable techniques for healing and balancing the body, mind and spirit.

Chapter Seven:
Mind, Body and
Spirit Connection

"Happiness is when what you think,
what you say, and what you do are in harmony."

- MAHATMA GANDHI

A peaceful state of mind, a balanced body and a sense of joy and happiness, all happening simultaneously, reflect a mind, body, and spirit in harmony. This is optimum health. There is no lack of guidance on how to create this condition. Let's first explore some of the Western healthcare options not mentioned thus far, options that can reduce stress and balance the mind, body and spirit.

According to research from the U.S. National Center for Health Statistics, a part of the Centers for Disease Control and Prevention, the American public spent $33.9 billion dollars on complementary and alternative medicine, or CAM, in 2007. That represents 11.2% of the 2.2 trillion dollars spent overall on healthcare, and money not claimable by health insurers. 22 billion dollars was spent on products such as fish oil, flaxseed, glucosamine and Echinacea. The other 11.9 billion dollars was spent on visits to acupuncturists, chiropractors, massage therapists and other CAM providers. In December of 2008, the National Center for Complementary and Alternative Medicine, or NCCAM, a part of the National Institutes of Health, or NIH, and the National Center for Health Statistics, released new findings on Americans' use of CAM. Approximately 38 percent of adults, or about 4 in 10, use some form of CAM. CAM is a group of diverse medical and health care systems, practices, and products that are not generally considered part of conventional medicine. The following therapies were included in the latest survey and will be touched upon in this chapter- homeopathy, naturopathy, chiropractic, osteopathic manipulation, and energy healing therapy such as reiki and massage.

Homeopathy is a system of medicine that has been around for almost 200 years and is based on the Law of Similars. Samuel Hahnemann, a German physician and "the father of homeopathy," worked on the principle that "similia similibus curentur" or "let likes be cured by likes." This meant that a patient's symptom was treated with a remedy that produced similar effects. For example, ipecac is a plant that can make you sick and vomit. As a homeopathic remedy, it is used to help someone stop nausea or vomiting. Homeopathic remedies are extremely diluted, administered in small doses, prescribed as a single remedy and dispensed solely when the patient's symptoms appear. The remedy can be a plant, mineral, animal or a chemical drug that is in accordance with the *Homeopathic Pharmacopoeia of the United States*, which is the official manufacturing manual recognized by the FDA.

Naturopathy is a holistic therapy that uses diet, exercise, massage and hydrotherapy to restore homeostasis within the body. This reestablished balance in the body allows for the curative "life force" to flow throughout the body, and prevents disease while maintaining health. The principle here is "let nature heal." Benedict Lust, a German doctor, founded the American School of Naturopathy in New York in 1901 and, to promote naturopathy, the American Naturopathy Association in 1919, and is considered "the father of U.S. naturopathy." In 1918, the philosophy of naturopathy according to Benedict Lust stated "the natural system for curing disease is based on a return to nature in regulating the diet, breathing, exercising, bathing and the employment of various forces to eliminate the poisonous products in the system, and so raise the vitality of the patient to a proper standard of health."

Chiropractic is a body therapy that concentrates on the adjustment and realignment of the vertebrae of the spinal column to restore the function of the central nervous system to balance the body. Chiropractic means "done by hands." In 1895, Daniel David Palmer pioneered the current chiropractic therapy. Before becoming a chiropractor, Palmer was a magnetic therapist, someone who uses magnets and electromagnetic energy to stimulate the body's "life force" in order to have it balance itself. Palmer was the first person to fix displaced vertebrae by using the transverse and spinous processes as levers. Chiropractors sometime use X-rays to help assess the spinal subluxations, or vertebral misalignments. Even Hippocrates understood the importance of a healthy spine and advised, "Get knowledge of the spine, for this is the requisite for many diseases."

Osteopathy is a healthcare modality that restores the body's normal mobility and function of joints and muscles by manipulating the body's structural framework. Osteopathy means "disease of the bones." Andrew Taylor Still, an American doctor, founded the study of osteopathy in 1874. Dr. Still believed that the musculoskeletal system played a major role in the vitality of a person. Osteopathy holds that by correcting problems in the structure of the body using manual techniques, known as osteopathic manipulative treatment, or OMT, the body is allowed to heal and enhance itself. Dr. Andrew Taylor Still opened the first osteopathic medicine school in Missouri in 1892.

Reiki is an energy healing system developed by Dr. Mikao Usui, in 1922. He was deeply meditating on Mt. Kurama, a sacred mountain north of Kyoto, Japan, when the information about this energy healing system was revealed to him. Rei is defined as "universal" and ki is defined as the "life force" in all living organisms. Reiki involves connecting the universal energy outside the body with the life force energy within the body. The Reiki practitioner helps to spread this healing energy by laying their hands on the patient's body in particular locations, such as the hips, shoulders and head. While attending graduate courses for Chinese medicine and working in the school clinic, a client of mine from the clinic asked if I wanted to study Reiki. The energy healing system seemed fascinating, so I managed to participate in the first two levels of training. The energy connection and boost was brilliant and powerful. I felt energized, centered and empowered to help more clients in the Chinese medicine clinic and in my personal fitness and wellness practice. My training handouts noted that the five principles of Reiki are:

just for today, do not worry
just for today, do not anger
earn your living honestly
honor your parents, teachers and elders
show gratitude to every living thing

Massage is another healthcare option that CAM surveyed. Massage improves blood circulation, detoxifies the lymph system, improves muscle tone and relieves stress. There are many types of massage but in this chapter, Swedish, acupressure and sports massage will be mentioned. Swedish massage has a therapeutic and relaxing effect and uses five techniques: long gliding strokes or *effleurage*, kneading or *petrissage*, rhythmic chopping or *tapotement*, rubbing or friction, and shaking lightly or vibration. Swedish massage has been credited to Per Henrik Ling, a Swedish physiologist and gymnast, who introduced this massage technique in Stockholm in 1812. After my fitness training business was booming, I decided that I needed to expand my wellness offerings so I attended a massage school for training in Swedish massage. The massage practice and training not only helped me provide better care for my clientele, it rejuvenated my own body.

Acupressure, or acupoint massage, is a type of massage that uses fingers to press key points on the surface of the skin, according to the theory and anatomy of Chinese medicine, to stimulate the body's natural self-curative abilities and create balance in the body. When the legendary sage Huangdi lived in China, this massage technique appeared in his book, *The Yellow Emperors' Classic of Internal Medicine*, or *Nei Jing*. Sports massage incorporates Swedish massage, acupressure and other deep pressure techniques to work on muscles, ligaments and tendons and includes resistance and isometric exercise movements during the treatment. Sports massage helps muscles recover quickly, increases flexibility and speeds up the healing process if there has been an injury. Sports massage was used at the 1924 Olympic Games in Paris. Runner Paavo Nurmi, the "Flying Finn" from Finland, won five gold medals at the Paris Olympic Games. He credited massage treatments as an important aspect of his training and the reason why he brought a massage therapist to the Olympic Games. Sports massage has been increasing in popularity ever since.

Massage therapies appeal to the body's sense of touch. But there are also Western healing treatments that can appeal to the other bodily senses of smell, sight, taste and hearing: these include aromatherapy, gemstones, metals and minerals, color therapy and music therapy.

Aromatherapy, by either inhaling or rubbing on your skin, gently activates your body's own healing energies and helps to restore balance to your body, mind, and spirit. The aroma comes from the essential oils of the bark, leaf, petal, resin, rind, root, seed, stalk and/or stem of the plant.

The Egyptians used essential oils for religious rituals, for deepening their meditative state, for embalming their dead and for everyday cosmetic use. The Greeks continued to value aromatherapy. Hippocrates emphasized the benefit of a daily aromatic bath and scented massage for good health. Dioscorides recorded aromatic and other plant properties while travelling as a military physician, in the book *De Materia Medica*, or *On Medicinal Substances*. In the 1920's, Rene Maurice Gattefosse, a French chemist, researched essential oils and their curative effects. While in his laboratory, he had accidentally burned his hand and on reflex, he immersed his hand in the closest liquid, which happened to be lavender oil. He was impressed by how quickly the burn healed without infection and without any visible scarring. In 1937, he wrote a book called *Aromatherapie: Les Huiles Essentielles Hormones Vegetales*, renamed Gattefosse's *Aromatherapy* when translated into English, and is credited with coining the word "aromatherapy."

Aromatic plants and herbs have been a part of Chinese Medicine since Shen Nong wrote the *Pen T'sao*, or *The Herbal*. This body of knowledge grew when Li Shizhen expanded the plant information in the encyclopedia *Bencao Gangmu*, or *Outlines of Roots and Herbs Studies*. Aromatic plants and herbs like *huo xiang*, or patchouli, dry dampness to improve digestion and prevent nausea. Other aromatics open the orifices and increase consciousness, like *bing pian*, or the processed resin of borneol camphor. This type of aromatic is used to treat convulsions or fainting.

The *Rig Veda* mentions aromatherapy, or *gandha chikitsa*, for Ayurvedic massage therapy or herbal medicine healing. The *Sharangdhara Samhita* contains important information about aromatics and the *Bhava Prakasha* describes aromatic plant characteristics. For example, a sacred herb *tulsi*, or holy basil essential oil, balances the mind, body and spirit and is an anti-bacterial, anti-viral and anti-fungal for the body. Another wondrous herb is Neem oil, or *azadirachta indica* oil, which reduces skin and scalp irritations such as psoriasis, repels insect bites and reduces inflammation from bites. Whether detoxifying or relaxing during a massage that incorporates aromatic oil with the treatment, drinking a cup of aromatic tea to help digest the meal, or rubbing aromatic lotion on the skin for cosmetic reasons, aromatherapy is up for the challenge.

Seeing beautiful gems, metals and minerals is pleasing to the eye and restorative for the body. In ancient Egypt, the brightly colored lapis lazuli and carnelian were popular gemstones for jewelry and artwork. The Roman emperor Nero used the gorgeous emerald to strengthen his eyesight. In the 1970's, some cosmetics used minerals, and in 1999, the Aveda cosmetic line added tourmaline to help the body look and feel beautiful. Currently, the precious metal platinum is being sought for healing. Two platinum-based anti-cancer drugs, cisplatin and carboplatin, are used in certain chemotherapy regimens. Western medicine continues to explore the value of gems, metals and minerals in its treatment repertoires.

Chinese culture not only values the aesthetics of gemstones, metals and minerals but, in addition, Chinese medicine has functional descriptions and purposes for items from each of these groups. The gemstone, metal and mineral characteristics are cold, cool or warm in temperature, heavy in weight, descending in direction, salty in taste and travelling to the liver and kidney meridians. Like aromatherapy, the medicinal uses of gemstones and minerals are written in the *Pen T'sao* and *Bencao Gangmu*. For example, tourmaline detoxifies, apatite speeds up the healing of fractures or broken bones and jade promotes longevity. Acupuncture needles can be made in gold or silver. Gold needles tonify and fortify while silver needles sedate and calm the body's energy.

Ayurvedic medicine describes gemstones, metals and minerals according to their taste, temperature and function. For example, gold has a sweet taste, a hot temperature and improves the skin and joints and boosts energy. Silver is sour, cold and relaxes the body. The tonifying aspect of gold and the relaxing aspect of silver are similar to Chinese medicine. Copper is pungent, hot and detoxifies. Wearing a copper bracelet reduces rheumatism.

The *Bhava Prakasha* mentions gemstones, metals and minerals. The preparation process for gemstones, metals and minerals is extensive and important for proper medicinal result. The gems, metals and minerals are first purified and then burnt several times, maybe even up to a hundred times, and converted to ash, or *bhasma*. Prior to each burning, the ash is processed with fresh herb juices to neutralize their toxicity. This is a very specialized technique and when done properly, has incredible healing effects.

One of the things that make gemstones, metals and minerals so appealing is their color. Color itself can have therapeutic qualities, so let's look at how our three different cultures have used it in their respective healing practices.

Western natural medicine uses color, or chromotherapy, to restore balance. According to this system, each color has a particular healing aspect. The color red is stimulating, promotes blood circulation and clears congestion. Orange relaxes muscle spasms and improves digestion. Yellow stimulates the nervous system, reduces arthritis and activates the lymphatic system. Green is cooling and calming and reduces insomnia. Blue is a blood tonic, builds vitality and reduces inflammations. Indigo purifies blood, is relaxing and promotes good muscle tone. Violet stimulates the spleen, promotes inspiration and aids in bone growth. The color may be recommended to wear as clothing or jewelry, or be painted on the walls of a special space used for meditating, or a therapist may use a specific colored light during a healing session.

In Chinese medicine, color is associated with the five elements. The wood element is associated with green, the fire element with red, the earth element yellow, the metal element white and the water element black. Colors are considered in herbal formulas or nutrition. For example, a black herb such as *shu di huang*, or radix rehmanniae glutinosae conquitae, is a kidney tonic. This herb tonifies the blood, and nourishes the yin, and can reduce palpitations, insomnia and night sweats. Color is also used in nutrition. Some examples are a pear, which is white on the inside, and helps produce fluids and lubricate dryness to reduce a cough from the lungs; or a watermelon, which is red on the inside, and reduces summer damp heat and acts as a cooling diuretic.

In Ayurvedic medicine, color is associated with the chakras and has various functions. The first chakra, or muladhara, is associated with the color red. Some of the functions for the color red are enhancing circulation, building blood and relaxing muscles. The second chakra, or svadhishthana, is associated with the color orange. Orange acts as a decongestant and elevates mood. The third chakra, or manipura, is associated with the color yellow. This yellow color improves metabolism, absorption and digestion of food. The fourth chakra, or anahata, is associated with the color green. Here, the color green can improve immunity, build muscle and reduce inflammation. The fifth chakra, or vishuddhi, is associated with the color blue; blue can reduce eczema and stress. The sixth chakra, or ajna, is associated with the color indigo. Indigo can balance hormones and increase tranquillity. The seventh chakra, or sahasrara, is associated with the color violet and is responsible for balancing neurotransmitters and creating bliss. The light from the color is absorbed and transmitted through the body's chakras and marma points.

Massage involves the sense of touch, aromatherapy the sense of smell, gems, metals and minerals the taste and sight sense, and color the sense of sight. That leaves one sense left to mention, the sense of hearing, which, in the healing systems under review, is experienced through music. With Western medicine, music therapy is the use of music by a healthcare professional to promote healing. Music encourages expression, increases social interaction and reduces symptoms of pain. Some research shows that music therapy decreases high blood pressure, depression and insomnia. Music therapy began during World War II to help soldiers reduce the effects of shell shock. In 1944, Michigan State University established the first music therapy degree program in the world. Music therapy patients might listen to sounds as varied as classical music, singing children, waves crashing on the ocean or birds happily chirping.

In Chinese medicine, the musical notes are associated with the five elements and use a pentatonic, or five-note, scale. The wood element is associated with the note *jiao*, the fire element is associated with the note *zheng*, the earth element is associated with the note *gong*, the metal element is associated with the note *shang* and the water element is associated with the note *yu*.

In Ayurvedic medicine, the chakras are regulated by sound and musical notes. The first chakra is associated with the sound *la* and the musical note C. The second chakra is associated with the sound *ba* and the musical note D. The third chakra is associated by the sound *ra* and the musical note E. The fourth chakra is associated by the sound *ym* and the musical note F. The fifth chakra is associated by the sound *ha* and the musical note G. The sixth chakra is associated by the sound *ah* and the musical note A. The seventh chakra is associated by the sound *om* and the musical note B. The Recreation Therapy-Rehabilitation, Medicine Department, Clinical Center, at the National Institutes of Health, in Washington D.C., has used a Thera Sound Music Table for healing. The Thera Sound Music Table allowed the body to feel the vibration and hear the sound and music to balance the seven energy centers, or chakras, in order to create a state of deep relaxation and release tension.

Identifying the causes of stress whether mental, emotional, physiological, spiritual, environmental, societal or cultural, hereditary based or family triggered, is also necessary when deciding a course of action to rebalance and heal the body. One way of identifying the sources of disharmony is to check your journal from Chapter Six and really analyze what you have written. Use that insight to make a positive change. One simple and healing approach is to write an affirmation to support what you have written. This will begin to create a positive solution.

Affirmation Diary

*Visit **vitalityfusion.com** to print a copy of the Affirmation Diary exercise and write your own personal affirmation. For example, if the hand you the least write with scribbled, "I am tired and useless." The affirmation to support your body might say, "I am full of energy and very important." Repeat the affirmation until your body feels an uplifting shift. After the affirmation reinforcement, some other options to balance your mind, body and spirit might be to take a bath with energizing bath salts or attend to the needs of those less fortunate, to offer service and be useful.*

I am full of energy and very important. I am full of energy and very important.

Conclusion

The ultimate goal for healthcare and medicine is a clear understanding of what constitutes health and wellness. One approach, used in this book's treatment of exercise, is to look at some combination of Western, Chinese and Ayurvedic health ideologies and techniques. Many of the ancient remedies are still as effective as when they were first applied, while the advancements in medical research have provided a better understanding of human mechanics and diagnostic and treatment protocols for illness. Rather than reflexively labelling many energetic or sensory therapies "alternative" or "new age" because they have not yet undergone enough proven scientific research and testing according to modern Western medicine, it is worthy to remember as a Philadelphia physician, Marc Micozzi, so poignantly states "what we call alternative medicine is traditional medicine for 80 percent of the world, and what we call traditional medicine is only a few centuries old." A better approach, and one that can be used as more empirical testing is being done, is to begin to integrate all the extant medicinal information, expand options for optimum health, and create an exchange of information similar to what existed during the ancient Silk Road or, in a more recent example, when Chinese and American doctors visited each other's countries to study medicine in the 1970's.

Another aspect to consider when designing a cross-cultural optimum healthcare model is how the ever-increasing spread of technology is rapidly connecting the world. With this increased sharing of information, one that recognizes few national boundaries, it is important to use all of our intellectual "know-how" in order to find a solution for optimum health and energy.

That "know-how," that intelligence, has come to be recognized as having a few differentiations. We now recognize "IQ" as academic intelligence and "EQ" as emotional intelligence, referring to the ability to be aware of our own feelings and those of others, and to manage those emotions. Psychologist Daniel Goleman helped to develop the information on emotional intelligence. The IQ and EQ are a combination of the multiple intelligences, developed by psychologist Howard Gardner, who listed them as linguistic, spatial, kinesthetic, logical-mathematical, musical, naturalist, interpersonal, intrapersonal and existential.

What is needed next, especially in the West, is to develop a better understanding of "SQ," or spiritual intelligence, and to incorporate it into our healing practices. Faith with a belief in God, truth and the divine wisdom, is essential for healing the body and planet. Studying and listening to nature rather than rejecting its information and healing gifts are critical to accomplishing this task. So first connect to God, feel the love and light, and with this, learn how to "lighten up." Next, listen intently to nature. Only then can a body's free will decide and act upon what is best for its mind, body and spirit. The body's senses can help awaken the insight to create the best balance no matter the cultural origin. Oprah Winfrey's last television talk show, in May of 2011, focused on her connection to God. She stated her success was "because nothing but the hand of God had made this possible for me." She also mentioned she knew she was never alone and that she listened for the guidance that she knew was greater than her mind. When she didn't listen, mistakes happened. She expressed that "God is love and God is life and your life is always speaking to you." This connection to God, that Oprah described, is our SQ, or spiritual quotient. The search for enhancing your IQ, EQ and SQ is not only of great value in terms of its teleology or goal, but the search itself becomes an intrinsically healthful way of living life.

One of the keys to achieving this health is to realize that our bodies become what we think, feel, eat and absorb. Fuel the body with fresh food and drink and feed your body with positive thoughts, feelings and energy. Live a life that has real moment-to-moment quality, not just one filled with a busy routine. There are many options open to each one of us in our search to achieve this quality; in fact, this book is actually a compendium of such options, surveyed across time and three different cultures. In attempting to have the reader interact with the material through exercises (or *Exaircises!*) at the end of each chapter, these options reveal just how useful they can still be, if only actively engaged. It is my hope that these pages have not just added insight into the vast intelligence and wisdom of our ancestors, but also opened a new unified path to optimal health for each one of us today.

Appendix

Here are some additional testimonials about Susan Shane and her *Exaircise* program from clients over the past two decades:

"*What I love and in fact is the best part, is getting results. The tension would quickly leave after Susan's treatment, I always felt refreshed and relaxed.*"

-NATALIE COLE, ENTERTAINER

"*Susan Shane is a tremendous therapist, one who has the ability to spiritually administer a healing of the body.*"

-MARY WILSON, THE SUPREMES

"*Two years ago I was in an accident. Both my arms and wrists were broken. Susan Shane's training healed my body and saved my sanity.*"

-BOB RAFELSON, DIRECTOR, "PUMPING IRON, FIVE EASY PIECES"

"*With her help I got off my back and could return to the racquet club.*"

-CLIFF LACHMAN, ASSOCIATE PRODUCER, "ENTERTAINMENT TONIGHT"

"*I recommend this program to anybody who has had bad results with traditional aerobics and weightlifting programs.*"

-JIM ZEIGLER, PRODUCER, "ENTERTAINMENT TONIGHT"

"Susan's method of exercising has changed my life. I am a healthier and happier person."

-SUSAN ROSS, PRODUCER, "LIFESTYLES OF THE RICH AND FAMOUS"

"Susan Shane is an extremely knowledgeable trainer who knows how to motivate."

-FONDA ST. PAUL, PERSONAL MANAGEMENT

"Her workout is safe, fun, and is changing my body fundamentally into the shape I want. I can't recommend it highly enough."

-SUE ANN LEEDS, ACTRESS

"The workouts are unique. They leave me feeling refreshed and energetic. And I look great."

-RENEE GOLDEN, ENTERTAINMENT ATTORNEY

"My work productivity and general outlook have improved. Most important, Susan has taught me how to release my stress and channel it out of my body. It's an excellent program."

-PETER LEVINE, ATTORNEY

"My mind and body are renewed with inner strength and a greater sense of well-being."

-JOY DAVIDSON, PH.D. "DR. JOY," PSYCHOLOGIST, AUTHOR

"For the severe arthritis in my back and hip, I tried everything: orthopedic help, nutritionists, chiropractors. But after a month with Susan Shane, I am almost free of pain and look forward to playing tennis again. Susan has incredible knowledge of how the body works."

-DR. VIVIEN L. GARY, PH.D.

"Susan is a consummate professional, reliable, dependable and gets the job done. Her techniques really work. You see results in a short time and in a fun, relaxing manner."

-DR. LILLIAN GLASS,

SPEECH, COMMUNICATIONS SPECIALIST

169

"Since I began working out with her body training, the differences in me both physically and mentally are astounding. Susan Shane's program is fun, easy to learn, and continues to give me a tremendous sense of accomplishment. It's one of the best things I've ever done for myself. I recommend it for everyone!"

-MIRIAM BASS, RETAIL EXECUTIVE

"We've enjoyed working with Susan Shane for over eight years. She is knowledgeable and expert in her techniques. Her approach is non-threatening yet positive and effective in her results."

-ELLY AND JACK NADEL, SANTA MONICA, CA

"I feel wonderfully firm and toned from these workouts. Now I welcome regular exercising."

-KATYOUN, SKIN CARE SPECIALIST, BEVERLY HILLS, CA

"As a personal trainer, Susan Shane brings knowledge about one's body. She has helped me gain strength and proper carriage, as well as conquer fatigue."

-JUDY FOSTER, HOUSEWIFE

"Throughout my 30 year baseball career, I've experienced many sports medicine programs. It wasn't until I worked with Susan for a couple of sessions and practiced her teachings for about two weeks, that my recurring leg problems for the past two years healed."

-STANLEY MARTIN, PROFESSIONAL BASEBALL PLAYER,

CALIFORNIA ANGELS, BALTIMORE ORIOLES

Initially, *Exaircise* was planned to be a book on its own. Here is a foreward written for that particular project.

"Ms. Shane has written an extremely interesting and versatile book about good health, and with a valid scientific approach.
I find her emphasis on diaphragmatic breathing especially useful for all readers who suffer with chronic fatigue and neurasthenia.

Diaphragmatic and abdominal breathing have always been part and parcel of traditional Chinese medicine. It promotes the circulation of qi, or breath of life, restores the electrical balances in the body, and revitalizes all the internal organs. This results in improved mental acuity and awareness, as well as building stamina for daily chores.

Ms. Shane introduces the importance of the concept of "mens corpore, mens sana"... a sound body, therefore a sound mind. The workout and conditioning exercises are simplified and easy to follow. I am especially fond of her spontaneous and joyous approach in imparting the message of her philosophy for fitness and better living to her readers.

This is certainly one of the most helpful and read-and-do-it-yourself books for fitness...in recent years."

DAVID K. YOUNG, M.D.
HOLISTIC AND PREVENTATIVE MEDICINE
ENCINO, CALIFORNIA

Bibliography

Adams, Kamryn. "Potency Vs. Efficacy." July 2011. <http://www.ehow.com/about_5533091_potency-vs-efficacy.html>.

Alphen, Jan Van and Anthony Aris. Oriental Medicine. Boston: Shambala, 1997.

"Alternative Medicine: Hope or Hype?" ABC News Turning Point. 26 Sept. 1996, Transcript #158: 10-11.

"Alternative Medicine Spending Soars." 24 May 2010. July 2011. <http://peoplebeatingcancer.org/blog-entry/alternative-medicine-spending-soars>.

Amber, Reuben. Color Therapy. Santa Fe, New Mexico: Aurora Press, 1983.

Ames, Louise, Frances L. Ilg and Sidney M. Baker. Your Ten-to-Fourteen-Year-Old. New York: Dell, 1988.

Anderson, Nina. "120 and Healthy! It's Common in the Republic of Georgia." July 2011. <http://www.manyhands.com/articles/georgia.htm>.

"Appendix A. Ayurveda's History, Beliefs and Practices." July 2011. < http://www.ncbi.nlm.nih.gov/books/NBK33781/>.

"Armenian Food and Culture." 2005. July 2011. <http://www.food-links.com/countries/armenian/armenian.php>.

"Atreya." Apr. 2011. <http://ayurport.com/Ayurveda/jsp/principles/atreyaPop.jsp?KeepThis= true&TB_iframe=tr...>.

"Atreya Samhita in India." 7 June 2005. April 2011.<http://www.india9.com/i9show/Atreya-Samhita-71143.htm>.

"Aveda History." Aug. 2011. <http://www.aveda.com/aboutaveda/history.tmpl>.

"AyurFoods, AyurFoods." July 2011.<http://www.ayurfoods.com/ayurveda-nutrition.php>.

Ayurvedic Institute. "The Ancient Ayurvedic Writings." 2002. July 2011. <http://www.ayurveda.com/online-resource/ancient-writings.htm>.

"Ayurvedic Mental Therapy for Ailments." 2009. Aug. 2011. <http://www.ayurvedic-medicines.org/ayurveda/mental-therapy-for-ailments.htm>.

"Ayurvedic View on Metallic Medicines, Ayurvedic Medicine for Heart Problems." Aug. 2011. <http://www.rejuvenateyourheart.com/ayurvedic-view.html>.

Balch, James F. and Phylls A. Prescription for Nutritional Healing. 2nd ed. Garden City Park, New York: Avery Publishing, 1997.

Bellis, Mary. "History of Vitamins." July 2011.<http://inventors.about.com/library/inventors/bl_vitamins.htm>.

Beinfield, Harriet and Efrem Korngold. Between Heaven and

Earth. New York: Ballantine, 1991.

Bensky, Dan and Andrew Gamble. Chinese Herbal Medicine. Seattle, Washington: Eastland Press, 1990.

Borysenko, Joan. Minding the Body, Mending the Mind. Cambridge, MA: De Capo Press, 2007.

Capacchione, Lucia. The Power of Your Other Hand. Franklin Lakes, NJ: The Career Press, 2001.

Chabner, Davi-Ellen. The Language of Medicine. Philadelphia: W.B. Saunders Company, 1991.

"Chakra Therapy-Balancing With Colors and Sound." 2005. Aug. 2011. <http://www.chakra-colors.com>.

Chan, David. "Chinese Nutrition by Food Group." Notes from Nutrition course. Santa Monica, CA.

"Chen Family Taiji." July 2011. <http://members.fortunecity.com/chentaiji8/history.html>.

Cheng, Xinnong, ed. Chinese Acupuncture and Moxibustion. Bejing: Foreign Language Press, 1987.

Cherry, Kendra. "Left Brain vs. Right Brain." July 2011.<http://www.psychology.about.com/od/cognitivepsychology/a/left-brain-right-brain.htm>.

"Chinese Creation Myths." May 2010. <http://www.crystalinks.com/chinacreation.html>.

"Chinese Medicine Chronology." May 2010. <http://www.shen-nong.com/eng/history/chronology.html>.

"Chinese Medicine History-Acupressure." July 2011.<http://www.

mcpt.com.au/acupressure.php>.

Colt, George. "See Me, Feel Me, Touch Me." Life Sept. 1996: 36.

Cooksey, Gloria. "Lust, Benedict (1872-1945)". 2011. July 2011. <http://www.findarticles.com/p/articles/mi_g2603/is_0007/ ai_2603000767/>.

Dalleck, Lance and Len Kravitz. "The History of Fitness." July 2011. <http:www.unm.edu/~lkravitz/Article%20folder/history.html>.

Dass, Vishnu. 2006. Mar. 2011. <http://www.bluelotusayurveda. com/dhanvantari_art.html>.

Deyo, Richard A. and James N. Weinstein. "Low Back Pain." 1 Feb. 2001. July 2011. <http:www.nejm.org/doi/full/10.1056/ NEJM200102013440508>.

"Dietary fiber: Essential for a healthy diet." Mayo Clinic. 19 Nov. 2009. July 2011. <http://www.mayoclinic.com/health/fiber/ NU00033>.

"Dietary Guidelines for Americans, 2010." July 2011. <http://www. health.gov/dietaryguidelines/2010.asp>.

"Different Types of Yoga." July 2011. <http://www.matsmatsmats. com/yoga/yoga-disciplines.html>.

"DNA Ayurveda The Vedas." Apr. 2011. <http:www.dnaayurveda. com>.

Douillard, John. "Timeless Wisdom for Getting Fit." Vegetarian Times. Apr. 1996: 80-89.

Dychtwald, Ken. Bodymind. New York: Pantheon, 1977.

"Emotional Intelligence/Daniel Goleman." 2011. Aug. 2011. <http://danielgoleman.info/topics/emotional-intelligence/>.

Ergil, Kevin and Jason Wright. "How do Food and Drug Administration CGMPs for Dietary Supplements affect Oriental Medicine Practitioners?" American Acupuncturist. Spring 2010: Vol.51: 28-31.

"Extraordinary Yang Organs." May 2011.<http://tcm.health-info. org/Zang%20Fu%20foundation/Extraordinary-Yang- organs.htm>.

"Francois Magendie: Biography from Answers.com." July 2011. <http://www.answers.com/topic/fran-ois-magendie>.

"Francois Magendie's Summary Physiology." July 2011.<http:// www.marshall.edu/library/speccoll/virtual_museum/hoffman/ magendie. asp>.

"Frequently Asked Questions- Massachusetts General Hospital, Boston, MA." July 2011. <http://www.massgeneral.org/bhi/faq/>.

Friedman, Aaron D., M.D. "Medicine." Academic American Encyclopedia. 1981.

"Galen of Pergamum." Mar. 2010. <http://campus.udayton. edu/~hume/Galen/galen.htm>.

"Gemstones-Precious Gems: The History of a Concept." Aug. 2011. <http://www.ganoksin.com/borisat/nenam/rw-1.htm>.

Gimbel, Theo. Healing Through Color. Essex, England: C.W. Daniel Company Ltd, 1980.

Gunther, Bernard. Energy Ecstasy and Your Seven Vital Chakras. North Hollywood, CA: Newcastle Publishing, 1979.

Halpern, Marc. "Ayurvedic Nutrition." July 2011.<http:www.

dreddyclinic.com/online_resources/articles/ayurvedic/nutrition.
htm>.

Haynes, Fiona. "The Lowdown on Low Fat." July 2011.<http://
lowfatcooking.about.com/od/lowfatbasics/a/fatlabels.htm>.

"Hellerwork-Henry Spink Foundation." July 2011. <http:www.
henryspink.org/hellerwork.htm>.

"Hellerwork Structural Integration." July 2011. <http://www.
hellerwork.com>.

"Herbal medicine: an introduction." July 2011. <http://www.
complemed.co.uk/herbalmedicine/index.htm>.

"Highlights of the U.S. Controlled Substances." July 2011. <http://
www.enotes.com/drugs-substances-resources/highlights-u-s-
controlled-substances-act...>.

"History of Aromatherapy." July 2011. <http://www.essentials-of-
aromatherapy.com/history_of_aromatherapy.html>.

"History of Aromatherapy." July 2011.<http://www.quinessence.
com/history_of_aromatherapy.htm>.

"History of Ayurveda." 13 Aug. 2008. May 2011. <http://www.
articlesbase.com/alternative-medicine-articles/history-of-
ayurveda-520578.html>.

"History of Ayurveda." Mar. 2011. <http://www.floridaediccollege.
edu/ayurveda/history.htm>.

"History of Ayurveda." Mar. 2011. <http://www.theholisticcare.
com/Ayurveda/History%20of%20Ayurveda.htm>.

"History of Chiropractic." World Chiropractic Alliance. July 2011. <http://www.worldchiropracticalliance.org/consumer/history htm>.

"History of Ida P. Rolf." July 2011. <http://www.rolfguild.org/idarolf.html>.

"History of Naturopathy." July 2011. <http://www.vaxa/com/history-of-naturopathy.cfm>.

"History of Osteopathic Medicine." July 2011. <http://www.aacom.org/about/osteomed/Pages/History,aspx>.

"History and Philosophy of Naturopathic Medicine." July 2011. <http://www.southbaytotalhealth.com/Naturohistory.htm>.

"History of Split Brain Experiments." July 2011.<http://www.macalester.edu/psychology/whathap/ubnrp/split_brain/Pioneers.html>.

"History of Sports Massage." July 2011.<http://www.thebodyworker.com/sports_massage_history.htm>.

Holstrom, John. "Ayurvedic and Chinese Medicine: Diagnosis and Constitutional Analysis. Seminar notes. San Diego, CA. 28 Feb. 2010.

"How to Calculate the Fat Percentage of Food." July 2011. <http://www.ehow.com/how_5701760_calculate-fat-percentage-food.html>.

"How to Read the New Food Label." American Heart Association brochure.

"Howard Gardner's Multiple Intelligences Theory." Aug. 2011. <http://www.pbs.org/wnet/gperf/education/ed_mi_overview.html>.

"Hundred Schools of Thought." New World Encyclopedia. 13 Dec. 2008. May 2011. <http://www.newworldencyclopedia.org/entry/Hundred_schools_of_thought>.

"Information on Ayurveda- History of Ayurveda." Apr. 2011. <http://www.kirlian.org/hinfo/chronoayur.htm>.

"Jack LaLanne-About Jack." July 2011.<http://www.jacklalanne.com/jacks-adventures/index.php>.

Jacobson, Michael F., Lisa Y. Lefferts and Anne W. Garland. Safe Food: Eating Wisely in a Risky World. Los Angeles: Living Planet Press, 1991.

Jaffe, Lynn. "Nixon, Appendicitis, and Acupunture." May 2011. <http://ezinearticles.com/?Nixon-Appendicits,-and-Acupuncture&id=2500342>.

"Joan Boryensko at Omega." July 2011.<http://eomega.org/omega/faculty/viewProfile/5c710abbdb969ddf39a2bea0cb7ec9c2/>.

"Joan Boryensko Bio." July 2011. <http://premierespeaker.com/joan_boryensko/bio>.

"John C. Pierrakos: Information from Answers.com." July 2011. <http://www.answers.com/topic/john-c-pierrakos>.

Jones, Kevin Lance. The Evolution of Chinese Medicine in East Asia. 1985.

"Kapila." Mar. 2011. <http://www.britannica.com/EBchecked/topic/311732/Kapila>.

Kemper, Cynthia L. "EQ vs. IQ-emotional intelligence, intelligence quotient." Aug. 2011. <http://findarticles.com/p/articles/mi_m4422/is_9_16/ai_57786889/>.

Lad, Vasant, and Anishe Durve. Marma Points of Ayurveda. New Mexico: The Albuquerque Press, 2008.

LaLanne, Jack. Fitness and Health Club training manual. 1984.

Lasagne, Louis. "Medicine." World Book Encyclopedia. 1985.

"Legend of the Phoenix and the Dragon." Jan. 2012. <http://www.holymtn.com/teapots/LegendPhoenixDragon.htm>.

Levitt, Shelley. "The Lowdown on Mineral Makeup." Aug. 2011. <http//www.webmd.com/healthy-beauty/features/the-lowdown-on-mineral-makeup>.

Life Science. Columbus, Ohio: Glencoe/McGraw-Hill, 2008.

Lindemans, Micha F. "Churning of the Ocean." Mar. 2011. <http://www.pantheon.org/articles/c/churning_of_the_ocean.html>.

"Lu Hui (aloe)." July 2011.< http://www.encognitive.com/node/14552>.

Manal, Naima. "Osteopathy Definition." July 2011.<http://www.ehow.com/facts_5507023_osteopathy-definition.html>.

Manilal, K.S. "Hortus Malabaricus." May 2011. <http://www.keralauniversity.ac.in/component/content/article/43-imagelinks/102-hortus-ma...>.

"Manu." Mar. 2011.<http://www.mythencyclopedia.com/Le-Me/Manu.html>.

Marani, Sara. "Quest Goes On For All-Round Platinum Cancer Drug." 2009. Aug. 2011. <http://www.cancerpage.com/news/article.asp?id=2907>.

"Massage Therapy." Natural Vitality Center of New York. July 2011. <http://naturalvitalitycenter.com/massage_therapy.htm>.

"Medicinal herb-Tulsi." July 2011.<http://ayurveda-foryou.com/ayurveda_herb/tulsi.html>.

Memmler, Ruth and Dena Lin Wood. Structure and Function of the Human Body. Philadelphia: J.B. Lippincott Company, 1987.

Mendes, Elizabeth. "In U.S., Frequent Exercise Rebounds Slightly in 2010." July 2011. <http://www.gallup.com/poll/146132/frequent-exercise-rebounds-slightly-2010.aspx>.

Miller, Richard C. "The Psychophysiology of Respiration: Eastern and Western Perspectives." The Journal of the International Association of Yoga Therapists. 1991: vol.2, no.1: 13-14.

Moore, Christine. "A Guide to Massge." New Woman. Mar. 1990:122-124.

"Music Therapy." 2008. Aug. 2011.<http://www.cancer.org/Treatment/TreatmentsandSideEffects/ComplementaryandAlternative...>.

Natural Health Handbook. Secaucus, NJ: Chartwell Books Inc., 1984.

NeemAura Naturals. July 2011. <http://www.neemauranaturals.com/>.

Ni, Maoshing A. Chinese Herbology Made Easy. Los Angeles: The Shrine of the Eternal Breath of Tao, 1986.

"NSGA Sports Participation in 2010 Survey Released." 9 June 2011. July 2011. <http://www.nsga.org/i4a/pages/index.cfm?pageID=4492>.

"Nutrition and Your Health: Dietary Guidelines for Americans." Appendix G-5: History of the Dietary Guidelines for Americans. July 2011. <http://www.health.gov/dietaryguidelines/dga2005/report/html/G5_History.htm>.

"Nutrition for Everyone: Basics: Protein." Centers for Disease Control and Prevention. 23 Feb 2011. July 2011. <http://www.cdc.gov/nutrition/everyone/basics/protein.html>.

"Nutrition Pyramid Nixed, USDA Launches New Plate Graphic." Huffington Post. 2 June 2011. July 2011. <http://www.huffingtonpost.com/2011/06/02nutrition-pyramid-out-new-plate-graphic_n_8...>.

"Opium Wars." The Columbia Electronic Encyclopedia. 2007. May 2010. <http://infoplease.com/ce6/historyAO836734.html>.

"Oprah: America's high Priestess- - The Washington Post." 26 May 2011. Aug.2011. <http://www.washingtonpost.com/blogs/on-faith/post/oprah-americas-high-priestess/2011/05/...>.

"Oprah final episode-The TV Column- The Washington Post." 25 May 2011. Aug.2011. <http://www.washingtonpost.com/blogs/tv-column/post/live-blog-oprah-final-episode/2011/0...>.

Osborn, David K. "Greek Medicine: Dioscorides." 2010. July 2011. <http://www.greekmedicine.net/whos_who/Dioscorides.html>.

"Paracelsus." 2009.<http://www.westerncultureglobal.org/paracelsus.html>.

Patrick, George. "The Effects Of Vibroacoustic Music On Symptom Reduction." Medicine Department, Clinical Center, NIH. Mar./Apr. 1999.

Pizer, Ann. "Yoga Style Guide." 13 July 2011. July 2011. <http://yoga.about.com/od/typesofyoga/a/yogatypes.htm>.

"Platinum." Aug. 2011. <http://www.unctad.org/infocomm/anglais/platinum/uses.htm>.

Plotnik, Rod. Introduction to Psychology. 2nd ed. New York: Random, 1989.

"Professor Li Chung Yun (1677-1933) 256 years old." 2006. July 2011. <http://www.crescentyouth.com/board/showthread.php?t=26431>.

"Publication of Surgeon General's Report on Physical Activity and Health." 12 July 1996. July 2011. <http:wonder.cdc.gov/wonder/prevguid/m0042984/m0042984.asp>.

"Pythagoras." July 2011.<http://9waymysteryschool.tripod.com/sacredsoundtools/idl13.html>.

"Pythagoras and Biosophy." July 2011. <http://www.iamuniversity.org/iamu/mobile/literature/lodges/western_esoteric_lodge/385-P>.

"Pythagoras of Samos." July2011.< http://www-history.mcs.st-and.ac.uk/Biographies/Pythagoras.html>.

Reddy, Bill. "Self-Cultivation- A Critical Element for AOM Practitioners." The American Acupuncturist. Winter 2009: Volume 50: 20.

Redmond, Michael. "Survey of Western Pharmacology." Notes from Pharmacology course. Santa Monica, CA. 1992.

Reston, James. "Now let me tell you about my appendectomy in Peking..." New York Times 26 July 1971. May 2011. <http://www.eastwestacupuncture.net/reston.htm>.

"Rise of Indian Nationalism". May 2011. <http://www.linkup.au.com/india/rise_of_indian_nationalism.htm>.

Robinson, Corinne H., Marilyn R. Lawler, Wanda L. Chenoweth and Ann E. Garwick. Normal and Therapeutic Nutrition. 17th ed. New York. Macmillan. 1990.

"Rolf Institute of Structural Integration." July 2011. <http://www.rolf.org/about/history>.

Schofield, Lina. "The Effects of Emerald Gemstone." Aug. 2011. <http://www.ehow.com/info_8429979_effects-emerald-gemstone.html>.

"Seasonal Balance." Ayurvedic nutrition handout. 31 Oct. 1996. Shaynebance. "History of Yoga- A Complete Overview of the Yoga History." July 2011.< http://www.abc-of-yoga.com/beginnersguide/yogahistory.asp>.

Shima, Miki. The Medical I Ching. Boulder, Colorado: Blue Poppy Press, 2001.

"Shiva." Mar. 2011.<http://www.mythencyclopedia.com/Sa-Sp/Shiva.html>.

"Sound Therapy." Aug. 2011. <http://healthalt.org/methods/descriptions/Sound%20therapy%20.php>.

"Split Brain Experiments." July 2011.<http://nobelprize.org/educational/medicine/split-brain/background.html>.

Stariell, Tarra. "Early Origins of Bioenergetic Analysis." 2003. July 2011.<http://www.thecenterforselfdiscovery.com/article-newearly.html>.

Svoboda, Robert E. Prakruti. Albuquerque, New Mexico: Geocom Limited, 1989.

"Swedish Massage at SpaFinder." July 2011.<http://www.spafinder.com/massage/swedish.htm>.

"TCM history- Modern China." May 2010.<http://www.shen-nong.com/eng/history/modern.html>.

"TCM history- The Ming Dynasty." May 2010. <http://www.shen-nong.com/eng/history/ming.html>.

"TCM history- The Qing Dynasty." May 2010. <http://www.shen-nong.com/eng/history/qing.html>.

Thiel, John E. Aerobics Theory and Practice. Sherman Oaks, CA: Aerobics and Fitness Association of America, 1985.

"Tulsi-Holy Basil." July 2011.<http://www.sacred-medicine.org/ayurveda/tulsi.php>.

"Types of Herbs and Healing Properties." July 2011. <http://www.legendsofamerica.com/na-herbs.html>.

"U.S. alternative medicine spend reaches $33.9 billion- July 31, 2009." July 2011.<http://blogs.nature.com'news/2009/07us_alternative_medicine_spend.html>.

"USDA Food Pyramid Gone: A History of Food Guides." Huffington Post. 2 June 2011. July 2011. <http://www.huffingtonpost.com/2011/06/02/usda-food- pyramid_n_870457.html>.

"Use of Complementary and Alternative Medicine in the United States." July 2011.
<http://nccam.nih.gov/news/camstats/2007/camsurvey_fs1.htm>.

Veith, Ilza. The Yellow's Emperor's Classic of Internal Medicine. Berkeley and Los Angeles: University of California Press, 1972.

"Vilcabamba-Longevity." July 2011. <http://www.vilcabamba.org/longevity.html>.

"Vishnu." Mar. 2011.
<http://www.sanatansociety.org/hindu_gods_and_goddesses/vishnu.html>.

Wallace, Adam. "Qigong and Traditional Chinese Medicine." Qi The Journal of Traditional Eastern Health & Fitness. Winter 1994-1995: vol.4, no.4: 11.

Wallach, Joel. "Dead Doctors Don't Lie." Cassette tape. Benson Promotions, Inc. 1995.

Wang, Yuan, Warren Sheir and Mika Ono. "Eating with the Seasons." Oriental Medicine. Winter 2010: 18,26-27.

"What are the medicines." Homeopathy Natural Medicine for the 21st century. 1993: 3.

"What is the History of Reiki?" The International Center for Reiki Training. July 2011. <http://www.reiki.org/faq/historyofreiki.html>.

"Wheeler-Lea Act." July 2011.
<http://american-business.org/858-wheeler-lea-act.html>.

Wild, Oliver. "The Silk Road." 1992. May 2011.
< http://www.ess.uci.edu/~oliver/silk.html>.

Wilson, Roberta. A Complete Guide to Understanding & Using Aromatherapy for Vibrant Health & Beauty. Garden City Park, NJ: Avery, 1995.

"Xia Shang Zhou Chronology Project." 5 March.2010. May 2010.
<http://en.wikipedia.org/wiki/Xia_Shang_Zhou_ Chronology_Project>.

"Yoga." Alternative Healthcare. San Diego, CA: Thunder Bay Press, 1997.

Yuen, Jeffrey. Notes from gemstone lecture. San Diego, CA. 2010.

Zeiser, Janet. Notes from Reiki I training, Aug. 1993, and Reiki II training, Sept. 1994.

Zhongjing, Zhang. Treatise on Febrile Diseases Caused by Cold. Bejing: New World Press, 1986.

Zhongjing, Zhang. Synopsis of Prescriptions of the Golden Chamber. Bejing: New World Press, 1987.

Index

Funk, Cashmir 79
fu organs 47
Fu Xi 19, 105

G

Galen 13, 14, 15, 35, 177
Gallup poll 101
gan 67
gandha chikitsa 158
Garcia D'Orta 36, 39
Gardner, Howard 166, 179
Gattefosse, Rene Maurice 158
Gattefosse's Aromatherapy 158
Ge Hong 24
Ghandi 37
Golden Mirror of Medicine 26
Goleman, Daniel 166, 177
gong 105, 121, 162
Good Manufacturing Practices 68
Grandmaster Chen Xiaowang 107
gunas 50

H

Hahnemann, Samuel 16, 154
Hammurabi 12
han 67
Han dynasty 23, 105
Harrison Narcotics Tax Act 65
Harvey, William 15
Hatha yoga 114
Heller, Joseph 143
Herbal Classic of Shennong 23
Hippocrates 12, 35, 63, 99, 155, 158
Hippocratic Oath 12
Homeopathic Pharmacopoeia of the United States 154

Qian Jin Yao Fang 24, 30
Qian Jin Yi Fang 24, 30
Qi Bo 19
qi gong 50, 105, 121
Qin dynasty 23
Qing Dynasty 26, 27, 30, 186

R

rajas 50
rakta 52
rasa 52, 95
re 67
reiki 154, 187
relaxation response 142
Reston, James 28, 30
Rhazes 14, 35
Rig Veda 34, 38, 69, 114, 158
Roentgen, Wilhelm 17
Rolf, Ida 143
Roman emperor Nero 159
Roosevelt, Theodore 65

S

sahasrara 53, 161
samadhi 114
Sama Veda 34, 38
San Jiao 49
sattva 50
se 67
Serturner, Friedrich 65
Seven Emotions 45, 46
shang 162
Shang Dynasty 20, 29
Shang Han Lun 23, 29
Sharangdhara Samhita 36, 69, 158

Yitian Ni 5
Yizong Jinjuan 26
Yoga 114, 115, 176, 182, 183, 185, 187
Yoga Sutra 114
yu 162

Z

Zang organs 47
Zhang Qian 23
Zhang Sanfeng 107
Zhang Zhongjing 23, 29
Zhao Xuemin 26, 30, 67
zheng 162
Zhenjin Dacheng 25
Zhenjiu Jiayiying 24
Zhen Quan 24, 67
Zhou Dynasty 20, 29
Zhu Peiwen 26
Zou Yan 22, 29

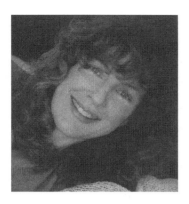

About the Author

Susan Shane graduated magna cum laude from Emperor's College of Traditional Oriental Medicine in Los Angeles and has been a licensed acupuncturist since 1994. She is also a Diplomate in Acupuncture and Chinese Herbology with the National Certification Commission for Acupuncture and Oriental Medicine. She holds a B.A. in Theater Arts and Dance and a 2nd degree black belt in taekwondo. Susan has participated as a long-standing member of the Community Advisory Board at the Scripps Center for Integrative Medicine in La Jolla, completed post graduate studies in gynecology with Dr. Yitian Ni and has been a wellness lecturer at college campuses and corporations, ranging from UCSD to Qualcomm. She has appeared on the American Entrepreneur segment of the Financial News Network and has been interviewed by *New Body*, *Men's Guide to Fashion* and *Mature Health* magazines. Her professional affiliations are with the American Association of Acupuncture and Oriental Medicine and the California State Oriental Medical Association; she has belonged to the National Sports Acupuncture Association, Aerobics and Fitness Association of America and the International Association of Yoga Therapists. Susan is passionate about teaching how to be vital and healthy, and currently lives with her husband, two children, and the family vizsla, Amber, in San Diego, California.

53032477R00118

Made in the USA
Lexington, KY
28 September 2019